Joan Lock has been a saleswoman, nurse, woman police officer, employment bureau interviewer, assistant librarian, advertising copywriter and airline clerk. Now resident in London, she is married to a Metropolitan police officer.

Please, Nurse!

JOAN LOCK

An Orion paperback

First published in Great Britain as *Reluctant Nightingale* in 1970
by J.M. Dent & Sons Ltd
This paperback edition published in 2013
by Orion Books Ltd,
Orion House, 5 Upper St Martin's Lane,
London WC2H 9EA

An Hachette UK company

1 3 5 7 9 10 8 6 4 2

A CIP catalogue record for this book is available
from the British Library.

ISBN 978-1-4091-2813-7

Printed and bound in Great Britain by
CPI Group (UK) Ltd, Croydon CR0 4YY

The Orion Publishing Group's policy is to use papers that
are natural, renewable and recyclable products and
made from wood grown in sustainable forests. The logging
and manufacturing processes are expected to conform to
the environmental regulations of the country of origin.

www.orionbooks.co.uk

To my mother

Contents

CHAPTER I   Prelude 1

CHAPTER II   The Real Thing 12

CHAPTER III   Theatre Going 24

CHAPTER IV   Smithfield 39

CHAPTER V   Stormy Nightingale 46

CHAPTER VI   Tempestuous Nightingale 61

CHAPTER VII   Fieldman–Duty Medley 74

CHAPTER VIII   Night-Duty Medley 87

CHAPTER IX   Mostly Wendover 101

CHAPTER X   Smithfield Revisited and Night Wandering 114

CHAPTER XI   Nightmare 129

CHAPTER XII   Migratory Nightingale 136

Epilogue 141

Acknowledgements

To Maureen, Dinah and my mother: grateful thanks for professional advice and assistance.

To my husband: for his help in editing this book and persistence in offering useful, though not always welcome, criticism.

CHAPTER I

Prelude

I had no intention of becoming a nurse. In fact I was determined *not* to be a nurse, mainly, I suppose, because it was expected of me.

'Have you got a vocation?'

or

'Going to carry on your mother's good work then?'

No I hadn't and I wasn't. What's more I'd never been even slightly interested. I was going to be something much more exciting. A journalist, that's what.

The Youth Employment Officer smiled patiently. Journalism was crowded, difficult to get into and needed *some* educational qualifications: a flair for English composition was not enough. For a girl fresh from secondary modern school it was impossible. I believed her. I couldn't bear the idea of an office, so all that seemed to be left for an ambitious but untalented child was shop work.

I spent three months on the haberdashery counter of a large store. Ugh. A year and a half in the haberdashery department of an even larger wholesaler's—not quite so ugh—and a week in a tiny, select men's wear shop where the proprietor swore at me for doing up parcels in the manner I had been taught in the wholesaler's. The Labour Exchange declared this impossible; the proprietor was a gentleman of the old school and known to them personally. Clearly I was no lady, and a liar to boot.

During this time I attended night school where I struggled half-heartedly with the complexities of shorthand and typing (I thought an office might be better after all) and found myself quite incapable of mastering either. I discovered boys as well, which didn't aid concentration. I was bored and unhappy but didn't know what to do next. Suddenly nursing didn't seem to be such a bad idea—worth a try, at least. But I was still only sixteen and a half and could not start my general training until I was eighteen.

The Penhurst Ear, Nose and Throat Hospital on the edge of Chessingham, the nearest town, had vacancies for Junior Assistant Nurses. So I said farewell to my few friends, who acted as though I was taking the veil and were quite sure that I would not be seen again. They were very surprised when I appeared a week later, on my first day off.

'Junior' was the operative word; we were simply skivvies and not allowed to do 'real' nursing, though when I look back I'm horrified that we were allowed to do any in our untrained state! But we were useful cheap labour, there was no doubt about that.

Via one of the fringe branches may seem like a gentle introduction to medicine. In fact it couldn't be bloodier. Not tragic but bloody. Even Out-Patients, where I commenced my (for the want of a better word) career, might have been specially selected for a gory initiation.

I reported in my American-style cap and shapeless white overall with starched belt (the accepted dress until one had been there long enough to warrant a proper uniform). But white suited me and, though nervous, I felt quite proud and pleased with myself as I passed the waiting patients.

There were two others on the nursing staff in Out-Patients. Stern, efficient Sister Collins and a thin, nervous, older woman with hennaed hair. The latter was a 'genuine' Assistant Nurse but it soon became evident that her prime function was to be despised by the 'proper' nursing staff (the S.R.N.s) who didn't know where she could have been trained. Only one consultant surgeon was on duty that day, so we both helped Sister. We shouted patients' names, ran hither and thither with patients' notes, washed instruments after use, etc. Though feeling a fraud when patients deferentially addressed me as 'Nurse', I wallowed in this new-found respect and looked suitably saintly when they whispered what a grand job we girls did.

The parade of cases was to become familiar: running ears, deafness, sinusitis, nasal polyps and deflected nasal septums. The deaf had tuning-forks held first to the front of their ears and then on the bone behind. I found the use of this instrument somewhat whimsical but it was apparent that to hear it behind the ear was most important. If the patient couldn't hear it the surgeon would shake his head sadly when asked hopefully for a hearing aid. But sometimes it was only wax which would be duly softened and syringed away.

Running ears were examined, cleansed and painted with gentian violet; the exotic effect belied the vile smell always associated with this complaint.

The first blocked noses were declared to be deflected nasal septums and dispatched for an admittance date to be arranged. Halfway through the morning the third blocked nose appeared on a very miserable young man. Mr Henry, the surgeon, declared this one 'sinus' and proceeded to dip long spills tipped with cotton wool into a mixture of cocaine and adrenalin. These he pushed up the young man's nose, two or three in each nostril. The effect was bizarre; he looked like the victim of some fiendish oriental torture.

'The cocaine is for anaesthetic and the adrenalin to reduce the bleeding,' Sister informed me. 'Put him back in the waiting-room, please.'

'Polyps,' muttered Mr Henry after examining the next

3

patient, so we made ourselves another of these stick creatures and sent him out to frighten the other patients too.

Five minutes later it was decided that the first victim was ready.

'We're going to pierce his sinus, Nurse,' said Sister, deliberately ignoring the fluttering Assistant Nurse. 'You can hold him—like this.' She placed her hands on his head. That looked simple enough. Mr Henry removed the sticks and grasped a pointed, steel tube-thing. He stood up, legs astride, in front of the patient, braced himself and pushed the frightening instrument up the man's right nostril. The head promptly went back and sharply to the left.

'Hold him still, Nurse,' snapped Mr Henry. The harder he pushed the more the man tried to draw his head away. I had, by now, grasped the idea that I was meant to resist this urge and keep his head firm. The surgeon pushed, I resisted. I was sure the awful pointed thing was going to plunge deep into the man's brain at any minute. Then I felt a sickening crunch. Mr Henry was through to wherever he wanted to go.

He stood back for a moment to regain his breath, then he leant forward and removed the inner portion of the instrument, leaving an outer tube in place. Water was then flushed through the tube and came out of the man's nose and mouth with a mixture of blood and infected sinus matter. Both surgeon and patient looked very pleased at this. I felt sick.

Then we did the polyps, which was worse, much worse, though our victim was remarkably cheerful throughout his ordeal.

'Nice to be cleared out and be able to breathe again for a while,' he smiled as I cleaned him up.

'Do they really come back?' I exclaimed, aghast.

'Oh yes,' he said, 'I have them done about once a year when they've grown good and thick!'

'I'll finish that,' said Sister, appearing at my elbow. 'You'd better hurry—you'll be late for first lunch.'

Our private lives were very much controlled. We were left in no doubt that we were a great trial and responsibility to the matron.

All we juniors lived in a large old house. Unless we had a late pass, which was not easy to get, we had to be in the home by 8 o'clock each evening. If we came off late shift at 8 p.m. we were required to sign in at the home by 8.15 p.m. This incarceration of young girls resulted in the bottling up of natural high spirits. Miss Frost, a middle-aged spinster, presided over this powder-keg.

Amongst the other eleven girls were my room-mate Simpson, an attractive girl with a ready smile and an easy-going nature; Burton, a jolly, fat girl; Heslop, who spoke in a pseudo-cultured manner about things we did not understand, to show that she was not common like us; Foxley, the devil who egged us on to commit heinous offences against discipline, then withdrew and adopted an innocent bystander pose; and Michaelson, who was attractive in a chubby way with her twinkling eyes and dimples but had exceedingly smelly feet. Fortunately, she was quite aware of the fact and her duty shoes used to spend the night resting on the top of the open window to freshen them up a bit.

Miss Frost found us difficult to control and her chief weapon was the threat of reporting us to Matron. An effective threat. One night Foxley and her room-mate decided that I should sleep in their bedroom as my room-mate was away. I declined, so Foxley implemented the decision by removing all my bed-clothes and taking them to their room. The two beds were then pushed together, all the clothes piled on and I was allotted the middle space. Much giggling ensued but was quietened when Old Frosty began to shout up the stairs.

We were drifting off to sleep when the castors moved, the beds parted and I crashed to the floor. Luckily I was relatively unscathed but a near-hysteria of giggling ensued. Suddenly we heard Miss Frost stomping towards us. The beds were quickly straightened and I was hidden under the middle lump.

When she burst in the other two were reclining innocently in bed. Foxley put on her charm, apologizing for the noise. She had dropped something on the floor. A little respect often placated Old Frosty and she knew Foxley was one of her good girls. She moved to go, but had a last word.

'You shouldn't put your beds together like this—look at these clothes.' She patted the lump that was me. A look of disbelief came into her eyes at the hardness of the blankets. She drew them back.

Chastened, we spent the rest of the night in our separate beds. Reported to Matron we were sure to be, despite Foxley's assurances that she would get round the old bat. But get round her she did. We all grovelled and gave promises to reform so Frosty postponed her decision, which meant she wouldn't report us.

Then she found the torn sheet—mine. Now she had no choice. She would have to tell Matron about the torn sheet. Finally the whole tale came out and the trivial incident was afforded the dignity of high drama in a manner which was to become only too familiar. Foxley looked hurt and wide-eyed and it became quite clear to Matron that I was a ringleader and a bad influence. I would have to be watched.

During the afternoon of my second day on Out-Patients, a white-coated porter dashed out of the adjacent theatre and up the stairs. In his arms he carried a small boy, held tilted so that his head was very low. Out of the little boy's mouth poured a stream of blood. I was horrified—there must have been some terrible accident. I ran to tell Sister.

6

She listened intently, then laughed. 'One of Mr Henry's T.'s and A.'s,' she explained.

It transpired that the child had just had his tonsils and adenoids removed. Patients from theatre were supposed to be taken up to the wards on trolleys and in the lift. But it was an old-fashioned lift which took ages to get anywhere. Hence, when Out-Patients was empty, the porters found it more practical to carry the T.'s and A.'s in their arms. It looked desperately barbaric but the child reached his bed more quickly and the porter could get back to the theatre in time to catch the next one off the conveyor belt. Also, the angle at which they were held gave a better drainage of collected blood from the mouth. So no one minded, as long as the public didn't see.

Whilst attached to Out-Patients I sometimes acted as skivvy to the theatre. Straightening deflected nasal septums seems a fairly civilized affair, but when it came to a mastoid, whom I was assured was very ill, the surgeon got out a hammer and chisel and banged away behind the unfortunate young man's ear. As the sickening hammering continued I thought: 'What's all that stuff about "the surgeon's slim, sensitive hands deftly searched . . ."?'

Usually there were at least half a dozen T.'s and A.'s on each list. They were removed in one of two ways. If large and nasty they would usually be dissected—in other words cut round and lifted out bit by bit and all bleeding points tied off as they went. The other method was to guillotine them. It did just that— chopped off their heads. The guillotine was a flat-topped instrument with a round hole in it, rather like a cigar cutter. The hole was placed over the offending tonsil and a flat blade pushed forward: chop or wrench, much blood. The obvious bleeding points were tied off and it was done. Some surgeons preferred to do more dissections; it was a matter of taste.

After three months in Out-Patients I went onto 'the wards'.

These were a series of rooms of varying size leading off a long corridor. The largest was the children's ward, which always smelled of a mixture of stale blood, anaesthetic and ice cream, especially on op. days. When children awoke from their T.'s and A.'s they had a rim of dried blood around their mouths and on their teeth. Later, hungry but complaining of sore throats, they were given ice cream and jelly to eat.

The trained staff on the wards consisted of two sisters, who were usually on alternate duties, and a staff nurse. The rest of the staff were us juniors. We wiped locker tops, served meals, emptied bedpans and held bowls while post-operative cases were sick.

Later I graduated to taking temperatures and pulses and even giving penicillin injections. I hated doing the latter and the men always complained that I hurt them. 'Nurse Waters is the best,' one would say and a discussion would ensue as to the merits and demerits of each nurse's style. I was to hear hundreds of such discussions over the next few years. I wanted very much to be liked and approved of, so when I found a sharp needle that went in easily without hurting I would use it over and over again. I don't think I was the only one.

I discovered early on that as well as being cheap labour we were cheap to feed. Food supplied was minimal. Scanty meals were supplemented with bread and jam but we were only allowed one pot of jam per week between the twelve of us. Food became an obsession—we seemed constantly hungry. Our wages covered our bus fares home, our black stockings (which we constantly snagged on beds), our outdoor uniforms and that was about all. Hence I was the envy of all when, towards the end of my stint as a Junior Assistant, I acquired Bill.

Bill was a plumber helping to build a power station about a hundred miles away. He came home some weekends. He was kind, quite handsome and very smartly dressed (northern men were not noted for their sartorial elegance). Easily the most sophisticated boy-friend I had ever had, he was rich with the overtime pay he earned. At weekends (when I could get time off) he lifted me out of the world of bread and jam and transported me to restaurants for meals, or to a hotel at a nearby resort where we drank exotic liquids at tables in the same room as we danced— just like on the pictures. The sweets and chocolates he bought me, together with food from home, staved off the worst of the hunger pangs during the week.

Our only regular serious cases were mastoids. Often admitted as emergencies, they could be very ill, but none died while I was there. Then one day came something quite new to me: a middle-aged man with cancer of the throat. His larynx was to be removed and he would never again speak normally. We were very sorry for him and gave him lots of embarrassed attention, but he was remarkably stoical.

When I returned from my afternoon break he was back from the theatre and very ill—at least by our standards.

'Nurse Driscoll, you will have to sit with him all the time,' said Sister. 'Take his inner tube out frequently and clean it. Should he start to choke or get worse, ring for me immediately.'

He was propped up on a backrest in one of the dreary little side-rooms. He looked awful. His eyes were closed, a tube from his nose was stuck onto his face with plaster and another tube carried blood into his arm. The mouth of a steel tube projected through the mass of bandages swathing his neck and gurgling sounds could be heard as he breathed—a tracheotomy.

I watched him like a hawk—how was I to know if he got worse, and what if he choked? The room was deathly quiet, apart from the gurgling tracheotomy tube. Every now and then I removed and cleaned the inner part as it became clogged with mucus.

9

Suddenly, despite my frequent attentions to the inner tube, the gurgling got thicker, his chest heaved and his face started to turn purple. I rang like mad. Sister raced in and applied the spout of the suction machine to his tube. The mucus soon cleared and he breathed easily again. After the fourth mercy dash it was decided that even an idiot like me could learn to point a suction tube at a hole, regularly, before he started to choke.

'But,' said Sister, 'you are to be very careful and don't forget to watch that drip as well.'

Careful—I was petrified. A life in my hands for the first time and I didn't like it one bit. I was glad to escape at 8 p.m., leaving my lonely vigil to the night staff.

Six months was enough of Penhurst, but not of nursing. Though not fired with a vocation (a term beloved of genteel ladies who will never get within twenty miles of a bedpan or sputum mug), I found it vastly superior to the dull alternatives I had previously experienced. Despite the awful hours and ridiculous discipline, it was still interesting and at times exciting. Most of all it gave me something which I desperately needed at the time: prestige.

My instant election to sainthood, even by friends who should have known better, was a very pleasant surprise. I also enjoyed the interest, friendly attitudes and good service at popular prices (or free) that I experienced in shops and on buses. At first I donned my outdoor uniform whenever possible but soon learned that this had disadvantages as well: the bore who leeched onto you at the bus-stop ('The surgeon said he had never seen an ulcer like mine before'), or the threat of an accident, resulting in my bluff being called in front of hundreds of people.

In private life the demand for instant diagnosis on the minimum of symptoms was trying. It was frightening how much faith people placed in the slightest information they could glean from a child like me, because I was 'in the know', as opposed to their fully trained, adult doctors who were obviously in a conspiracy against them.

I was now almost seventeen and a half and eager to commence proper training. I found that St Margaret's, a fair-sized hospital in the city, would accept girls six months early and without any educational qualifications. So St Margaret's it was.

CHAPTER II

The Real Thing

St Margaret's P.T.S. (Preliminary Training School) was neat, bright and modern. The single-storey building was separated into two areas, lecture and tutor's rooms in one and nurses' lounge and bedrooms in the other. I had never had a room of my own before, so I delighted in its pristine neatness and privacy. It was really a characterless box of the type to be found in most nurses' homes, police section houses and international American hotels. But this was my first encounter with the human battery cage and I was well satisfied.

Most lectures in the initial three-month course were on the duller 'grounding' subjects of anatomy, physiology, histology, hygiene and the simpler nursing procedures. Hygiene was excruciatingly dull, but the knowledge gained has proved invaluable. If something is amiss with your sewage farm or your waterworks is not working, I'm your woman. The advantages and disadvantages of sash and casement windows I'll throw in for free.

Anat. and phys. was a greater trial: so many complicated names had to be committed to memory. Bones were the worst—every bump, notch and line had to be learned. For instance, one side of the femur consisted of: head, great trochanter, quadrate tubercle, gluteal line, popliteal surface, intercondyloid notch, adductor tubercle, articulating surface for tibia, linea aspera, spiral line and small trochanter. That was just one side (the posterior aspect) of one bone! I found this minutiae of little value in practice.

Some of the names stuck because of their incongruity or whimsicality. Who could forget the romantic Islets of Langerhans and mysterious Ducts of Wirsung in the pancreas, or the sinister sino-auricular Node and Bundle of His in the heart?

We progressed to cells and tissues—'transitional ephithelium is a compound, stratified ephithelium'—and my poor, atrophied brain seized up altogether. I couldn't work up any enthusiasm for compound, stratified ephithelium or plain, non-striated muscular tissue.

As well as the usual skeleton we had lots of odd bones that could be slapped in our hands with the command 'Describe that bone'. But my favourite was a gaily coloured creature made of some sort of composition whose purpose was to display his viscera, muscles and blood vessels. Like a television announcer, he had a head and trunk but no legs. All his pretty organs lifted out and many of them took apart for inspection. A large, sectioned ear and an eye, layered like a giant aniseed ball, completed the anat. and phys. set.

Gerty was the poor relation of this set-up. Made of waterproof cloth and stuffing, she represented homo sapiens when incapacitated and had to suffer such indignities as repeated mock enemas, blanket baths, catheterizations, back rubs and a bed that was in a continual state of upheaval. What's more, she was always being accused of wetting her draw sheet and having to have it 'pulled through'.

I liked bandaging and was good at it. I derived pleasure from transforming a 'wound' into an aesthetically pleasing creation with repeated patterns evenly spaced. Making a neat divergent spica for an elbow or ankle was a challenge and doing all the fingers of one hand a joy. I'm glad I didn't stay to see the advent of the tubular bandage.

Even the simpler nursing procedures were dogged by medicine's insistence on the original Latin or Greek names and its members' longing for immortality. Hence bleeding from the nose was *epistaxis* and the only spectacle frame catheter carrier (for oxygen) in general use was the Tudor Edwards spectacle frame catheter carrier. Embellished names were useful for differentiating between the many types of one particular object, such as urethral catheters, but I didn't think there was any excuse for such verbal indigestibles as the Boothby, Lovelace and Bulbulian nasal oxygen mask. It was inevitably shortened to the B.L.B. nasal oxygen mask but we still had to know what the initials stood for.

Nonetheless, the instruction and running of the school was of a high standard and the staff did its best to make the dull and sometimes idiotic subjects more interesting; it wasn't their fault that application of leeches and cupping were still on the curriculum.

The threat of weekly tests kept us up to scratch, though one of the students seemed to have found a simple way out of them. Several times Jane complained of severe migraine and was excused. This maddened the rest of us. We didn't like her much anyway; she was always miserable and grumbling. She did have occasional cheerful spells when she would try to right her image, but we weren't having any and she was avoided.

Soon after going on the wards Jane went sick again. We wondered what she was trying to avoid now. There were further investigations and a new diagnosis: a brain tumour. Her headaches had been genuine and even her unattractive personality was probably due to the tumour. We swore we would make it up to her. But Jane died.

The uniform was one of the perks. Blue and white striped dresses, white starched collars and aprons and ridiculous but flattering butterfly caps. It improved our looks and made us feel like real nurses. I never tired of the romantic cloak with its dramatic scarlet lining.

The caps were a problem. They were fairly simple to make once you had got the hang of them (the swooping butterfly had to be created by hand from an unpromising oblong of starched cotton), but there was a knack in producing a snappy shape at the back and the right-sized perky front. Balance was important. A too large and heavy rear, even if perfect, would pull the front up and one would be fighting continually to keep it on. The trouble was, if one had a couple of tries and failed, the cotton began to look like an old dish-rag and final victory was impossible. A couple of the girls could always be relied upon to produce a 'good cap' at first go, so their services were much in demand.

Black stockings were a constant drain on our purses and even here personality played a part. They varied from sheer and sexy to opaque and frumpy. The sheer were more extravagant both in initial outlay and wearability, but the girls who wore them were more likely to get further pairs bought for them by susceptible males, so in the long run they were probably more economical.

As one of the *élite* who had done some nursing, I already possessed an outdoor uniform and flat black shoes so did not have that expense. We 'experienced' nurses stood out because of our aplomb, the way we knew it all already and by being distinctly unimpressed by the tales of gore. But this stance could prove tricky if the others took it seriously and expected us to know all the answers.

There were three men and thirteen girls in our P.T.S. The men lived out, thus avoiding much of the stringent discipline. Outstanding amongst them was Frank, who was tall, almost aggressively masculine and married. He assimilated information much more easily and enthusiastically than the rest of us. His know-all manner was only made bearable by his good humour and willingness to explain patiently complicated details to us simpler souls. To the Principal Tutor I've no doubt that he was 'one of those'— always thinking up absurdly complicated questions to try to catch him out.

Jenny, a trained nursery nurse, was the prettiest girl in class— almost beautiful in fact, although not so much in features as in texture and colouring: dark brown hair, liquid brown eyes and a fabulous complexion. Her girlish gaiety and easy-going nature quickly made her popular.

Barbara, though plump, short and not particularly attractive to look at, had lots of personality and was fun. She had led a most interesting life which she described vividly. Everything seemed to have happened to her and apparently men threw themselves at her in the most extravagant manner. We felt dull by comparison.

Martha had been brought up on a farm. In appearance she was like most country girls: not the dew-fresh, pretty perfection of the butter-ad girls, but rather coarse and unkempt. I well remember her immortal words oft repeated at the lunch table: 'Don't like this dry feeding.' Soon after we went on the wards, she returned to her livestock and presumably gave them wet feeding.

Helen, a blue-eyed blonde, did regular battle with Frank for his position at the top of the class. But this didn't stop her having a crush on him, which was not surprising since he was a strong, masculine figure and she a sensitive (though outwardly inde- pendent) orphan whose only family ties were sisterly. She wanted more than anything (and any of us) to be a good nurse and devoted herself to this end.

I moved the oddments on the locker and wiped where they had been. Nurses don't dust—that scatters evilly intentioned germs about. They wipe. I was doing a few hours on the wards to get the flavour and to supplement the theory we had learned at P.T.S.

As I continued to the table, I gave the occupant of the bed a friendly smile in passing. He didn't respond. Come to think of it he hadn't moved since my first approach. I had a good look at him. His eyes were half closed. Like most of the men in the small ward he was having a mid-morning nap. He certainly needed it. Looks very ill and emaciated, I thought, savouring one of my newly acquired words. Most uncomfortable way to sleep though. Sitting up supported by his backrest was normal, but he was leaning forward slightly, like a puppet with the wires relaxed, and his Tudor Edwards spectacle frames had slipped forward and a little askew on his nose.

Actually, he looked rather odd. Didn't seem to be breathing. No, a ridiculous thought. People don't die like that without anyone knowing or without a last few words! I knew it didn't have to be as dramatic as on the pictures, with the hero gulping out a nicely rounded, succinct sentence before his head fell decisively to one side. But it couldn't be this casual. Besides, no one else had noticed that anything was wrong and they knew the man. Deeply asleep and breathing very shallowly because he was so ill, doubtless. I hesitated. I could take his pulse. No, I'd look a right Charlie disturbing his nap like that. I was being dramatic.

I avoided looking at him again, finished his table and moved on to the next locker. The owner was a pleasant-looking young man of about thirty. He looked rather hard at me, then at the old man, and then back at me. The ward had been quiet when I came in but now I became aware of an air of expectancy. I looked up and saw that the eyes of all those awake were fastened on me, waiting.

The young man cleared his throat. 'Don't you think you'd better have a look at Mr Franks, Nurse?' he asked politely. 'He doesn't look too good.'

'Who?' I asked and blushed. My eyes followed his pointing finger.

'Oh yes, I didn't notice,' I lied.

I took a better look at him this time. It was obvious to anyone that there was something wrong, I thought, now that I was backed by a second opinion. I grasped his wrist and felt for his pulse. I couldn't find it. I searched but still none. Oh dear, I might be grasping too hard again; as he was so ill his pulse would be feeble. Lightening the touch did not help.

He felt cold and I couldn't see any sign of breathing. He slipped forward a bit more at my touch and his glassless wire spectacles were hanging grotesquely in mid-air. I pushed them back on his nose and made for the door, holding myself in check so as not to agitate the other patients—'a nurse only runs in cases of fire or haemorrhage'.

Once out of the door, I felt such niceties unnecessary in this dire emergency and made towards Sister at an unseemly scuttle. I was guilt-stricken. Perhaps my pride and tardiness had prevented him being snatched from the jaws of death and it would be on my conscience for ever. Murderess!

Sister was talking earnestly to a girl from X-ray when I panted up. Seeing my rather wild eye, she paused: 'Yes, Nurse?'

My words tumbled over each other. 'Mr Franks, Sister. I think he's dead!' I exclaimed dramatically. I waited for the startled response, followed by swift, efficient action. I got neither.

'Oh, is he?' she said. 'Thank you, Nurse. Put the screens round him will you? I'll be along in a minute,' and returned to her conversation. I was dazed and turned slowly away. Sister looked up again. 'Oh, Nurse . . .'

'Yes, Sister?' I asked hopefully.

'Don't run.'

'No, Sister.'

I didn't know what to do when I'd put the screens round, so I hid behind them with the body and started to worry as to whether Sister had heard me correctly—perhaps she hadn't understood—I was inclined to gabble. She arrived looking

18

crisper and more untouchable than ever. She removed her cuffs, briefly examined Mr Franks, then turned off the oxygen cylinder.

'Yes, you were right, Nurse—he's dead,' she confirmed.

Then she remembered my inexperience and smiled. 'I thought he would go this morning. It's a happy release for him.' She paused, then confided meaningfully, 'He was W.R. positive you know.'

I looked suitably impressed but wondered what she meant.

'He had a syphilitic heart,' she explained.

My imagination ran riot. How had syphilis got to his heart? I thought it was confined to 'those places'.

'You can help Nurse Bates to lay him out after Doctor's been. Good experience for you.'

'I have to go to lunch soon,' I stammered, feeling ungrateful. 'I've got to be back at P.T.S. this afternoon.'

'Oh, what a pity. Still, there'll be plenty of other opportunities.'

'Damn!' said Nurse Bates when she heard the news. 'We're behind as it is and it's almost lunch-time. I hope you've finished those lockers!'

The late-pass problem was becoming intolerable and the warden had now refused to allow us the key for the classroom part of our building, which meant no access to the electric ring specially installed so that we could have a hot drink before retiring.

We protested strongly to the tutors. They felt (understandably) they had no authority over the warden and suggested our only recourse was to see Matron. When it came to selecting the delegation, I learned an important lesson in my young life. I had thought it would be more effective to go mob-handed. Everyone had been staunchly behind militant me in this fight against petty tyranny. Suddenly, when it came to the crunch, there was a hasty withdrawal. Eventually a nice, sensible, older girl and myself went to see Matron. I was spokeswoman. Matron was sympathetic, in a difficult position (the warden was a retired matron), but would do what she could. We got access to the electric ring and more late-passes. *I* became notorious as someone who'd dared to go to Matron with a complaint before I'd even left P.T.S.! A trouble maker.

I certainly chose the wrong room, I thought bitterly, as I heard a gentle tapping on the window for the second time that night.

'It's unlocked!' I shouted. 'Help yourself!'

The window was opened noisily from the outside and bits of arms and legs intruded into the room.

'Give me a hand, then,' said a plaintive voice.

'Go to hell,' I growled. 'I'm not getting out of bed again. From now on everyone helps themselves.'

There ensued much grumbling, grunts of effort and dire warning of impending tragedy but I didn't budge. Finally, the whole body issued into the darkened room and grumpily stalked off to bed.

The doors were locked at 10 p.m. and, even in these more enlightened days, one couldn't get late-passes every night. True, we took turns to hold the key, but the entrance was opposite the old building and the warden had eyes and ears like a hawk. My room could not be seen by the warden. What's more, there was a short, L-shaped wall just to the right and almost level with my window. Great for sneaking in late, I thought when I first saw it.

I imparted the joyful news to my colleagues. At first I conscientiously assisted any latecomer to make the rather difficult ascent. Often a boy-friend gave support and encouragement at the other end. It was all good fun. But it soon got beyond a joke, as rather than go through the then usually pointless routine of trying for a late-pass, the girls would rely on my window and me.

I began the rather dodgy procedure of leaving the bottom window slightly open and making them help themselves.

It was our last night in P.T.S. and most of us were a little the worse for the imbibing of South African sherry. One of my climbers had not attended our little party, the other had left with her passionate boy-friend so that he could see her home properly —round the back. I was just settling down for the third time that night when I heard a noise under my window. It was a swishing sound, as if someone were walking round and round in the grass. I knew all the girls were in. 'Who's that?' I shouted. No reply. I listened hard. The noise had stopped. My imagination, or a cat, I decided.

I was nodding off when it started again, very soft but definitely discernible. A strange sound. I switched on the light to frighten off the possible prowler and because I had a horror of anything happening to me in the dark. It stopped again. I was beginning to heave a sigh of relief when I heard the unmistakable sound of a foot scraping the top of the wall. My curtains were open and my windows unlocked! He must be looking at me now!

I yelled, rocketed out of bed, through the door and into one of the rooms across the corridor. Here I found three of the girls talking. They were keeping each other company because they thought they had heard noises outside and were scared.

We formed a posse, opened my window and peered out, but saw nothing. There was no telephone in the building. To contact the warden it was necessary to cross in the dark to her house— and no one fancied doing that. Anyway, our misdeeds might come to light. Never mind, he couldn't do us much harm if we stuck together. We would report a possible prowler the next morning.

Except for a couple of brave souls who thought it all nonsense, the rest of our wing doubled up in the rooms on the opposite side of the corridor. As long as we were not alone we felt quite safe and it became a giggly adventure.

I was dozing off yet again when Jean burst in from the next room. 'Quick, something's happening to Helen!'

I regarded her sleepily, wondering where I was. Jean looked incomplete and defenceless without her glasses, I mused.

'Come on!' she yelled, and the urgency in her voice rocketed me out of bed once more.

Helen was on the floor having violent convulsions. I was stunned. Others were beginning to crowd into the room and eventually someone stopped being stunned for long enough to say, 'Something to put between her teeth.'

That she had already bitten her tongue was evident from the flecks of blood amongst the bubbling saliva around her mouth. We found a pencil but that was discarded as being too flimsy. A teaspoon was the only other suitable object to hand, but we had great difficulty getting her mouth open. Eventually, we prized her clenched teeth apart and risked our fingers inserting the spoon.

She promptly clenched her teeth again and bent it double. We saw that it might do more harm than good so withdrew it when we had the opportunity.

The convulsions gradually lessened in violence. Three of the girls had grabbed a torch and, prowler or no prowler, dashed over for the warden.

When the convulsions had abated Helen passed into the third stage, which often takes the form of mental confusion and some-times violence. Helen reverted to childhood. Before our astonished gaze, this girl, whose normal personality was of a slightly cynical, intelligent maturity far beyond ours, lapsed into lisping baby talk, coyly hugging her knees and happily rambling on about something her big sister had done.

Our minds had scarcely adjusted to this latest surprise when they were shattered by a piercing scream from the other wing.

22

We raced across to find a near-hysterical girl leaning on the wall, outside one of the toilets. When she became coherent, we gathered she had been enthroned therein when a hand appeared on the drainpipe outside—a man's hand.

The girl was somewhat worse for the sherry and inclined to the dramatic anyway, so some were of the opinion that she had been carried away by all the commotion and was a victim of auto-suggestion. But she seemed genuinely upset.

The warden arrived, quickly followed by an ambulance which took the unfortunate Helen to the hospital. A search of the grounds was conducted by the fearless warden but no intruder found.

We were all very concerned about Helen. She wanted so much to be a nurse and this incident, we felt, could prevent her attaining her ambition.

We straggled back to bed to grab a couple of hours' fitful sleep. Soon we would be doing *real* nursing, and wouldn't that be exciting?

CHAPTER III

Theatre Going

Our three months' training over, we were assigned to wards. Mine turned out to be the theatre. Blood and guts, it seemed, was to be my lot. I didn't mind, although it seemed a back-to-front way of learning the trade and thus a little confusing.

The theatre suite was of modern design and well-equipped. Twin theatres were approached through their own small anaesthetic rooms and connected in the middle by the sterilizing room and sluice, with its long row of basins. Doctors' and nurses' changing-rooms completed the suite.

I thought the theatres attractive with their spotless, pale green tiled walls, cream composition floors and gleaming chrome. Which was just as well because the spotless and gleaming bit was where I came in. But, to be fair, only the most senior student nurses' escaped the cleaning.

The start of the day followed a set pattern. We divided as nearly as possible into two groups: one for each theatre. There could be anything from two to six of us. Everything washable was washed with an antiseptic solution: walls, trolleys sinks, operating table, stools, bowl carriers and the huge, retractable centre-lamp which I thought the most beautiful and impressive thing in the theatre and loved to clean.

Then the anaesthetic room, checking the equipment as we went. Finally the surgeons' room, making sure the boots were clean and plenty of white hats, shirts and trousers were available.

The senior nurses, with perhaps a sister, were selecting and sterilizing the instruments for the first operations and supervising the endless autoclaving (sterilizing by super-heated steam under pressure) of towels, gowns, gloves and swabs.

The basic cleaning completed, we donned caps and aprons and went for coffee. In the dining-room I would greet any member of my P.T.S. like a long-lost sister. Even those with whom I had had little in common became soul-mates and we would huddle together comforting each other and comparing notes on how we would never make nurses. I was particularly isolated as most of the other girls had a classmate on their ward. Frank and Barbara were the only ones who didn't seem to need comforting.

Frank was as confident as ever, even appearing to have his presence acknowledged by the senior nurses with whom he chatted and laughed as if he were their equal. Barbara was still full of bounce, having lots of adventures, proving invaluable to her ward sister, noticing symptoms that had escaped everyone else's eye and averting tragedy by her prompt actions. This upset us a little because we were so obviously not valuable to anyone and if we acted promptly it was always wrong. But she was always so friendly and liberal with her good advice that we forgave her.

Sometimes I saw my mum in the dining-room. She was on Fieldman, the general surgical ward. No, not as a sister, as a student nurse. My mother had been a Registered Fever Nurse for more than twenty years. But lately, when working as a District Nurse, she found that not only did she receive considerably less remuneration than the S.R.N.s, but also her prospects of any rise were nil. Both her children had left home—my brother had joined the R.A.F.—so she determined to use this opportunity and 'take her General' at last. Mum was a few months ahead of me and was required to do only a two-year course, but nonetheless it was a fairly unusual situation, mother and daughter being

25

student nurses together. She also had an unusual privilege: she was allowed to live at home.

Back in the theatre battle would commence. Glamour went by the board when we put on the hair-concealing white bandana, white wellingtons, baggy theatre gowns and nose-tickling masks. Few girls could manage to bring a touch of individuality to this get-up, though some tried to soften the look and were always being told to 'Get that hair tucked in'. I must admit I found it pleasant to sink into anonymity at times.

At first I just watched but after a while was allowed to do some of the simpler setting-up jobs such as the sterile glove and gown trolley (making sure I had the correct size gloves for each member of the team). Also I was allowed to lift the large steel bowls from the sterilizers and place them in their stands, without touching the stands with the bowl-lifting forceps (Harrison's of course). This was no mean feat, as the bowls made a heavy, ill-balanced load and their curved lip was difficult to grasp. Deafening bangs and crashes often accompanied my first efforts and as if to emphasize my clumsiness the bowls would spiral, clang, clang, clang, on the floor. Most embarrassing during an operation when I ruined the surgeon's concentration.

Once on their stands, antiseptic tablets were placed in the bowls, then boiling water was poured upon them, the outside of the jug never touching the inside of the bowl. They were used mainly by the surgeons for rinsing the powder from their gloves, or the goo if they got too messy during the op.

Then into the anaesthetic room to take over the first patient, with his notes, from the ward nurse and await one of the two regular anaesthetists.

At first I had regarded the giving of anaesthetics as fairly simple until I saw young doctors having a go in emergencies. They always fussed, looked worried and had to suffer the surgeon's complaints about a blasted rigid abdomen (muscle-relaxing is part of the job).

The regulars were Freddie Johnson, who was large, paunchy and lascivious, and Dr Bruce, who was Scottish, rather nice-looking, conscientious and very circumspect. Both were natural and pleasant, with none of the remoteness or exaggerated sense of dignity to which many of the surgeons and some of the younger doctors were prone.

Dr Bruce was always kind and would quietly explain all his actions as he went along, without being patronizing. Freddie, whose lasciviousness was amiable, open and indiscriminate, would leer at me. All he could see were my eyes so he commented on them: 'Ah, the blue-eyed beauty today, I see! Pull your mask down, dear, you don't need it up in here. Mustn't spoil my fun.' He even managed to make 'Hold his arm for me' sound suggestive. But he was very good with the patients and his non-chalant air inspired confidence.

Pentothal injection into the vein, then gas and air from the anaesthetic machine, via a B.L.B. mask, to continue and deepen the anaesthesia. Freddie would slide the endotracheal tube neatly into the patient's throat, with the help of a laryngoscope, then attach it to the tube leading from the machine.

Whatever you thought of Freddie, you couldn't say he didn't know his job and do it with the minimum of fuss. Some of the nurses said they didn't see why they should put up with him and would do something about it one of these days but I, and most of the other juniors, were grateful for someone who didn't look through us as if we were non-existent, or become impatient at our fumbling inefficiency. In return, we were quite prepared to put up with his vague pats in the general direction of our bottoms. He rarely made it to our behinds anyway. Cloaked as they were in blue and white ticking and voluminous theatre gowns, exact location and identification was difficult.

Besides, he put the porter in his place. We didn't like the porter. He was a small, red-haired man, efficient enough but a know-all, who despised nurses and seized every opportunity to catch us out. Even more unforgivable, he was always right. In the anaesthetic room he would rush to assist the doctor, showing us how it should be done. But Freddie wasn't having any; he liked his nurses, blundering or not, and would say sharply, 'It's all right, Nurse can manage!', much to our glee.

The trolley and the heavy anaesthetic machine, with its anti-static chain tinkling on the floor behind, were towed into the theatre and the patient was lifted onto the table. The surgeon and his assistant were scrubbing-up by now.

We dirty nurses (or sometimes just dirty me) began to dash around trying to be where we were needed most; tying the assistant's gown, checking with Sister (who was scrubbed-up and busy behind her barricade of sterile trolleys) on the number of swabs in a newly broken pack, immediately chalking the number of swabs on the board, tying the surgeon's gown, getting a new pair of gloves for the assistant who had ripped the first pair, holding up the notes for the surgeon who suddenly decided that he wanted another look, uncovering the patient and finally removing the 'prep' dressing. Doing all of it with dispatch and *never* touching anyone or anything sterile with your dirty self.

At the first op. there would be several of us; we had nothing else to do, but as the list went on we would disperse to sluice, wards and sterilizing room.

The surgeon painted the exposed area a bright, inappropriately gaudy orange-pink, then chucked the swab and forceps on the floor, making a half-hearted effort to hit the bucket. Dressing towels were laid on and the initial incision made. Whenever I saw the horrible thick layer of globuled yellow fat just under the skin of an obese person I would vow never to become even plump, but of course I have—well, well-covered anyway.

With the op. now commenced, we settled down to a steadier tempo. When in the theatre and not in the sluice, swab count was my principal job. All discarded gauze swabs and the larger muslin packs were thrown on the floor or in the bucket, to be picked up by me; I ascertained the number in the blood-matted mass, then hung each one individually on a large pegged rack. Sometimes an assistant in a good mood would aim at me with a second swab when I was bending down to pick up the first.

I also checked and chalked up any new packs broken by Sister and kept an eye open for the needs of the anaesthetist, who might want to set up a drip, or require another endotracheal tube. If it were Freddie, he would be keeping an eye open for me and it didn't do to inquire of his needs.

A more experienced nurse would attend Sister's needs— fetching obscure instruments or a certain type of suture. But sometimes, if we were short or half staffed, as in the afternoon or evening, the senior nurse would be setting up in the sterilizing room. I would have to translate what I could make of Sister's whispered request, which had been issued through a mask and at a distance of about three feet (across a trolley, with me keeping far enough away to prevent my baggy gown touching its flowing drapes). Since I did not know the names of even the simpler instruments or the dozens of other accoutrements and was slow to learn, this could be a nerve-racking business. Especially if the whole op. had been suspended to await the execution of my errand. Sometimes the nurse had to ask Sister again, while I stood and looked stupid. Even more nerve-racking was to be left all alone with Sister and be forced to find the described object myself.

In between swabs I was usually handed a dish containing the bit that had been removed (a portion of stomach, a growth, stones or even a limb flopping in a bucket) to put in a safe place in the sluice. I never felt very squeamish about actual ops., but found that colour films shown in the P.T.S. of an op. or the birth of a baby would turn my stomach!

I never saw anyone faint in our theatre, mainly because of the business-like atmosphere, everyone having an important job to do and the absence of spectators. Dental surgery was occasionally performed on our patients by visiting dental surgeons and I found this more distasteful than major surgery. The patients were only lightly anaesthetized and thus moved and made gurgling noises through the blood. They were too obviously living people: I preferred the inanimate object.

Atmosphere varied with each surgeon, but generally was only tense when things went wrong, such as the patient ceasing to breathe or the surgeon accidentally nicking the liver. But if we opened an abdomen only to find it inoperable because of an extensive cancer growth, a huge depression would settle over the theatre; we felt that it would have been better if we hadn't looked and then it wouldn't have been there.

One surgeon kept a tense atmosphere all the time, merely by having an unpredictable and explosive temper. He was liable to throw things and had even been known to tip the contents of the hand bowl all over the floor when he found it did not contain his chosen solution. (Laymen are inclined to imagine there is one method only for doing things medical but in truth all doctors and surgeons have their pet methods and ideas and can be as temperamental as prima donnas if their instructions are not followed to the letter.) *He* acted not as though the particular antiseptic solution was not *quite* right, but as if it were sheer poison, even though every other surgeon in the hospital used it. Almost everything he used was different in some way from those used by other surgeons, but he was brilliant in his field and surgeons came from abroad to watch him operate.

Mr Prentiss, who had a gentle, friendly manner, used to ask Freddie how Alice was and mention that Edna was only saying the other day that it was time Alice and Freddie came over again. He would ask the latest arrival in theatre whether they had heard the cricket score. Endlessly patient but inclined to be pernickety, he finished off everything himself, right down to the impeccable row of skin stitches, and would even try to help with the dressings. He was fiction's surgeon: dark, lean and aesthetic looking, with slim sensitive hands and long fingers. Before the incision was closed, he insisted on a couple of puffs of penicillin powder to help prevent infection. None of the other surgeons used it and some considered it caused adhesions—but that's medicine.

Mr Eggleston (isn't it daft the way a 'Mr' works to become a 'Dr' then works even harder to become a 'Mr' again, which he was in the first place?) was withdrawn and undemonstrative. He expected efficiency, but was not given to wild, emotional displays if he did not get it. His cold anger was more dignified and just as effective, especially if he accidentally got a repaired glove —the patches 'come off in the wound'. There was little idle chat at his ops. and, though some of his patients complained about his abrupt manner, he was a very good surgeon. Most of the nurses agreed that they would like him for their big op.!

Mr Lane's temper was variable. It could be hearty and jovial or bluff and unreasonable. He looked like a farmer: chunky, red-faced, with stubby, square-shaped hands. His list was always quickly dealt with and with no nonsense. He had few obsessions and always left his assistant to 'close up'.

Our bone man, Mr Cartwright, was something of a favourite. Tall, lean and gangly, he had the vague, distracted air of a dedicated man, with no time for false pride. He had a reputation for being absent-minded about anything that did not affect his work. Stories, such as how he had driven somewhere and then walked home, having forgotten he had gone by car, were legion. His Friday mornings had an air of barely controlled hysteria and we all loved them. With patients positioned in each anaesthetic room and theatre, he would dash from one room to another, grunting and perspiring as he manipulated bones and joints, inspected limbs after removal of plaster, instructed how he wanted the plaster put on and sometimes applied it himself. Many of the patients were relatively healthy and awake, which was a change.

We followed his rather wild figure (not quite straight eyes fronted by plain spectacles, black hair awry, matched by tufts sprouting out of his white theatre shirt, which was never quite tucked in or buttoned-up properly), madly trying to keep up as he whipped through the motley crowd of people with plaster chests or rigid necks like Frankenstein's monster, children with their legs in frog-like plaster casts, and owners of arms and legs which had become mobile autograph albums (curious habit that).

His op. lists were also strenuous affairs. He started with the smaller stuff, removal of cartilage and straightening of bunions, then worked up to the full-scale productions such as replacing damaged hip bones with new plastic ones, spinal ops., amputations and pinning of serious fractures. These usually called for the presence of a large theatre staff, the plasterer and an X-ray girl with her huge mobile machine ready to take a picture to see if the pin was correctly in place or check the new hip action before closure.

Much of it reminded me of my father's work as a carpenter, as did the instruments, which included mallets, wrenches, chisels, nails, drills (power and hand), screws, screwdrivers (automatic and plain), rasps, braces, pliers, nuts and bolts, awls, spanners and saws (wire, circular and plain). Sawing through a bone during an amputation was one of the few things that *did* turn me a bit.

Mr Cartwright's obsession was sterility—a good one for a bone man, as infection can cause disaster. He was fanatical about it. The only object exempt from his insistence on impeccable sterility was his long nose. Apparently it breathed out sterile air, as it always peeped over the top of his mask (actually, he had to keep it out, or his spectacles would have steamed up). The trouble was, he did perspire so. Perspiration poured down his face and hung threateningly on the end of his nose as it was poised over a wound. This would force him to turn around and say 'Wipe'. Sometimes there was no one near enough and he loathed wasting time.

Once he turned and said 'Wipe' and I thought his wonky eyes were looking at me, but my colleague was equally sure they were looking at her. We collided in front of him, almost causing disaster by 'touching' him. If the slightest real or imagined touch occurred he would immediately strip off his sterile clothes and re-dress, even at the most involved point in the operation. After our collision a full-time wiper stood a few feet behind him at all big ops.

Inevitably, the patients are inanimate objects to those in the theatre. The nurse who assisted the anaesthetist may have chatted to them when they arrived from the ward but the rest of the staff never saw them conscious and they soon became completely anonymous under the towels. As far as we were concerned the patient was a laparotomy, gastrectomy, nephrectomy or appendicectomy and first, second or third on the list. He was also a rubber balloon on the anaesthetic machine, which caused concern and a possible hold-up when it ceased to inflate.

When everything was finished except the closing-up there was a pause. Sister counted her swabs, I counted mine, and we tried to make up a set. If there were any missing we were held up until we found them. Sometimes, in spite of my care, I had hung two on one peg or forgotten the one the anaesthetist had used for the drip and everyone would look peeved at my stupidity. Sometimes one would be hidden under the surgeon's foot or, despite protestations to the contrary, still inside the wound and everyone would laugh. But it was usually right first time. Sister also had to check her instruments whilst I kept count of any that had fallen on the floor, or had come with the stomach that had been handed to me.

All layers were then sewn up and the dressings applied in the surgeon's pet way. One used clips, another one long-stitch which was woven in and out just beneath the surface of the wound, leaving a tail at both ends. The latter did not leave such bad scars, but hurt like hell when it was taken out. One surgeon did not believe in dressings at all, but covered the stitches with a loose dressing towel, yet another had the latest see-through dressings, and Mr Prentiss had his couple of puffs of penicillin.

Now the surgeons enjoyed a short lull and a chat as they stripped off and strolled into the other theatre. Our work started again in earnest. Towels were cleared from the body and buckets and trolleys moved out into the sluice, to make way for the patient's trolley. The blanket pack was placed over the patient and the patient was lifted onto the trolley. Once he was out of the way, we got down to the cleaning again. First we picked up gloves and gowns from trolleys, hand-bowls and the floor. Some doctors just let them drop where they stood, and we would mutter 'Come the Revolution!' For them to put them on the glove trolley did not really make much difference to us physically, but it seemed a lot less arrogant.

We mopped the floor, wiped the blood stains from the furniture, tidied and re-stocked the anaesthetic room, reset the gown trolleys and filled the hand-bowls.

Then into the sluice to do the real cleaning. First the instruments, dishes and bowls were washed, as some of them would be needed again shortly, then all the bloodied dressing towels, muslin packs and gowns were put into one of the huge sinks of cold water. We rolled up our sleeves and got stuck in.

At first I was loath to let my fingers or arms touch huge lumps of slimy clotted blood and bits of tissue but I soon got over that in the perennial anxiety to keep up. Gloves were washed and hung to dry; when we were not too busy we played childishly with them, filling them with water so that they became bloated and grotesque.

By now the next op., if a short one, would be almost finished.

I liked it when Sister said, 'You take this patient to the ward, Nurse'. I always enjoyed this little trip as I dodged some of the tedious clearing-up and was able to see the wards. They seemed so animated and full of untidy life after our pristine and well-ordered domain.

The patients, and any odd visitors who might see us en route, were patently awed by my nun-like figure, as I held the patient's chin, vomit bowl and notes with one hand whilst steadying the bottle of blood with the other. Slipping down my mask, I would look serious and dedicated yet a trifle distant, as though I had seen things that I would not care to talk about but was carrying on bravely regardless. No one knew that I was a novice and that the porter despised me, except when he shouted instructions at every opportunity, always pleased to have someone timid and unsure to bully. When I got to my third year, I told him to mind his own business, to get on with his portering and to leave medicine to those trained to do it, which made him go purple with rage. For a long time, however, I was as apprehensive of him as of a surgeon.

Halfway through the list there would be a break for tea, unless the surgeon was one of those who always worked right through— which meant we had to as well. During the break an assistant might wander out to ask if we had that stomach or spleen or whatever; he would peer at it and maybe dissect it. Sometimes he took it back for the surgeon and himself to play with while they sipped their tea.

I found theatre work exciting, if a little impersonal. One never knew what would come up next and everyone felt involved and quite important at times. But my ego was frequently crushed as, being a slow learner, I was nearly always cast as the village idiot.

On Sundays we did more basic cleaning and tidying, folded swabs, filled drums, puffed gloves full of air and held them to our faces to detect pin pricks which we promptly sealed, whilst Sister tried to drum the names of the instruments into us. But sometimes, without warning, everything in this seemingly trivial scene could be shoved aside and the pace would quicken as we prepared once again to patch up a 'perf.' (perforated stomach ulcer) or reassemble yet another victim of man's aggressiveness on the roads.

I was Mr Cartwright's wiper. It was a long, gruelling operation near the end of a long list. The pin had been put in place, X-rayed, but was not quite right and a lot more cursing and messing about ensued. It was very hot and everyone was tense and tired.

Mr Cartwright raised himself from his curled-up position almost inside the wound, turned round to me, leaned over and, without taking his hand off his work, said: 'Wipe, please.'

Obviously he begrudged having to stop even for a minute at this crucial moment, but the sweat was starting to hang from the end of his nose and was in danger of falling into the wound. I wiped quickly and carefully, trying not to touch his gown and the sterile sheets or knock off his spectacles.

'Better do the glasses while you're at it,' he muttered.

A weirdly intimate thing to do, this, especially with the whole surgical team suspended in mid-action and watching as though hypnotized. Shaking, I removed, wiped and polished the spectacles and successfully completed the return journey to his ears. Relieved, I took my arms away but as they reached my sides the dreaded cry, 'You touched me!' thundered accusingly round the theatre.

My sleeve must have touched his gown. Everyone, especially me, was transfixed, as in a tableau. The spell was broken by Mr

Cartwright who furiously handed his instruments to his assistant and stamped away from the table, stripping off his gloves as he went. I ran to undo his gown. The other dirty nurse was already picking a clean gown out of the gown drum with the Cheatles forceps. I ran to the glove drums—no nines—his large size were always in short supply. My heart in my mouth, I rushed into the sterilizing room.

'Nine glove drum?' I yelled at the senior nurse.

'One drum used, the other, in the autoclave, got forgotten. Be out in five minutes.'

'Oh no!'

Sensing the panic, Sister had emerged from her barrier of trolleys and followed me into the sterilizing room, holding her arms, palms turned inwards, up to her chest like a kangaroo. She was rather dour but never panicked.

'Go and get the nines from the glove trolley in there,' she intoned slowly, indicating Theatre One. 'Take your time and *don't* drop them.'

Picking up the nearest Cheatles, I dashed into Theatre One, drew aside the protecting towel and picked up the gloves. As I got them airborne over the side of the trolley they started to slip. Trembling, I pushed them back over the trolley and dropped them. I slowed down and made sure I had them this time. Long journeys, carrying sterile items on forceps, were always fraught. We dropped things every day when they were only being moved two feet, so a long walk cut one's chances of safe delivery by half.

Holding them high, I made my way across Theatre One, through the sterilizing room where a wide path had been cleared for me, and into the other theatre. Everyone watched my progress around the operating table and giant X-ray machine. The blasted forceps began to slip again, but the waiting Mr Cartwright snatched the glove-packet out of my hand before I reached the trolley. He was beside himself with impatience to finish the job. Gloves on, he stalked back to the wound.

I was glad of the mask which hid my blushes but wanted to get away to the toilet and cry. As I stood there, thinking of my humiliation, tears began to well into my eyes. Dr Bruce wandered over as if nothing had happened and asked me to get another bottle of blood, though he didn't really need one yet.

Eventually, the protracted operation finished. Mr Cartwright leaned back exhausted, then turned round, stripping off his gloves once again. He glanced at me as I went to undo his gown.

'Now, Nurse, you can touch me all you want,' he joked and everyone relaxed and laughed.

CHAPTER IV

Smithfield

Mr Arthur, a strapping, six-foot-two policeman, was making a terrible fuss over getting out of bed. Oh, the pain. The visible effects of his meniscectomy (cartilage removal) seemed puny, compared with the afflictions of those around him, but the invariably athletic men who underwent this operation were frequently voluble about their suffering. Either a meniscectomy was really painful or strapping men were not stoical, I mused, as I whipped the sheets and blankets to and fro in unison with Nurse Sinclair, my partner in the daily bed-making ballet.

After two months on Mr Cartwright's ward I was getting quite slick at beds, though this wardful could never achieve the soldierly symmetry so beloved of matrons. Each bed presented a different outline. Mr Harper's had a four-poster frame supporting pulleys and weights which suspended his right leg in mid-air. The next bed sported a rounded bed-cradle, like a miniature Nissen hut. Mr Snelling, opposite, had a nice smooth bed but his arm, frozen in a wave or halfway to a salute, spoiled the silhouette. Sticks and crutches by the beds and the continual upheaval caused by the physiotherapists added to the chaotic appearance.

I was very lucky to have been transferred to Smithfield, the orthopaedic ward. It had a happy atmosphere and was quite different from any other, due to both the aforementioned chaos and the fact that most of the patients were younger than the hospital norm (their presence there usually resulting from accident rather than degeneration). So the majority were not really ill in the accepted sense of the word and were therefore quite cheerful and indeed patient. Except Mr Harper.

Mr Harper, a tall, athletic young man, was the victim of a motor-cycle accident. He had a fractured femur which was now under traction. His leg was proving a so-and-so to heal and he was restless with inactivity. We were not without sympathy for him, trussed up like this for a couple of months. In fact, we had a great soft spot for him, but he refused to accept his immobility and kept trying to do things that are physically impossible in a tilted bed and with one leg hung high in the air. We would hear the bed creak, see the heavy weights swing and dash across to catch him leaning over getting things out of his locker cupboard rather than submit to the indignities of being helpless.

Mr Desmond was sitting self-consciously by his bed, waiting to go home. He was scrubbed, shining and almost unrecognizable in his neat blue suit and dove-grey cap.

Seeing a patient in his day-clothes was always a shock; he assumed a different identity, as money, taste and position were now brought to the fore. Comforting for some, less so for others. That Mr Desmond was a miner was now clearly announced by the cap and the white silk muffler—they really do wear them. Pyjamas are a great leveller; only personality, voice and face count. Personality mostly. Dignity is the hardest quality to maintain.

We stripped Mr Desmond's bed and took away his locker to be cleaned. This increased his feeling of not belonging. He had been dispossessed and wandered over to sit stiffly by Fred's bed. Their chat was strained, though only yesterday they were casual muckers. Anyway Fred obviously wanted to listen-in on his earphones.

Then we did Fred's bed. Yes, he would like his back rubbed, he said a trifle too eagerly. I worked a lather of soap and water into the skin, then a brisk application of methylated spirits followed by talc, and a playful but smartish slap to finish.

He jumped and laughed. 'Lovely, Nurse, thank you. Wish you would teach the other nurses how to do it.'

I had the reputation for being the best back-rubber—the only one who put a bit of guts into it. Now there was an achievement!

Edna Lambert, a pleasantly attractive twenty-three-year-old, was in a room by herself. She greeted us cheerfully as always. Suffering from a T.B. spine, she had already spent a couple of years on her back in the Infectious Diseases Hospital and was now transferred to us for an operation. But that was not the end of her trials; she was to go back to the other hospital for a further long stay.

Edna and I had had a great rapport since I had done her 'prep' shave. I was required to shave her back and was somewhat apprehensive. Mr Cartwright was a stickler for a perfect shave, especially for a spinal op. My only previous experience was on a leg and a man's arm, both of which had been obviously hairy. I couldn't find any hair on Edna's back, only the most infinitesimal down, and I wasn't sure whether I should spend ages trying to remove it all, thus risking Staff's wrath for being a slow-coach. Neither did I want her to turn into the original hairy woman when it grew again. Eventually, she and I decided that the down must go. She was very patient with my amateur scraping and as I scraped we chatted.

She told me that she had been about to be married when she fell ill. After the doctor had explained to her fiancé the nature of the illness and that she would require a long stay in hospital, he promptly walked out, without seeing her and saying goodbye. She had neither seen nor heard from him since. We became great friends and I loved to go in and see her. Being a long-term patient she accepted nurses as people so one could drop the saint-like, ever-competent, angel of mercy pose that the other patients expected.

'Here,' she said as soon as I entered, 'have you seen the new houseman? Dishy!'

'Not bad,' I admitted, 'but married.'

'Oh, what a shame,' she murmured thoughtfully. 'I had him all picked out for you. Still, he does have cold hands.'

Nurse Sinclair wore her slightly disapproving expression—that sort of talk was not professional, but she looked sad as we closed the door. She was soft-hearted. She and I were supposed to look alike and had been mistaken for each other several times before we had even met. I couldn't see it and found it rather disturbing to be mixed up with someone else—after all I was unique! True, we were both fair-skinned, blue-eyed and had high cheek bones, but I had light auburn hair whilst hers was blonde. Her nose was classical while mine was anything but. Not that it was an insult to be mistaken for Nurse Sinclair. She was intelligent, pretty, efficient and a devoted nurse, full of kindness and—rare amongst nurses—a genuine sympathy for the patients. Nonetheless, it irked me a bit—she was obviously so much nicer than I and I felt that I suffered in comparison. Though I did think her a bit prissy and prudish, I never said as much; it would have seemed like sour grapes.

The main women's ward was bunged up with trolleys and screens—preps in progress. So we left it till last and went into the children's ward. If the patients looked odd in the adult wards they looked even odder here.

Simon's legs pointed straight up in the air, suspended by cords and pulleys. June, a blue-eyed fair-haired little girl, had her trunk and legs in a frog-plaster (shaped like a frog's back-legs), which was part of a long process to correct congenital dislocation of the hips. More common in blue-eyed, fair-haired little girls! The feet of three other children were fixed in various unnatural positions—outwards. They had talipes (club feet).

Whenever we could spare any time we wandered into this ward

to play with the children. Even so we had to be very careful. The extra but uninvolved adult attention made some of them very precocious.

Roger popped his head round the door. 'Get a bed ready in Two, Pott's fracture coming straight up from casualty.'

Roger was a second-year nurse. Very efficient and witty, though sometimes caustic. His blue-eyed, fair-haired, good looks attracted some of the girls, but although he had desultory little romances he seemed content to be gossipy friends with them.

We had just finished the bed when the Pott's came in.

'Last minute as usual,' complained the porter.

'Get lost,' said Roger, or words to that effect.

The injured man had a cushion pinned over his foot and ankle, not tightly but effectively giving support. Poor man, I could see why they thought it kinder to send him straight up to the ward and leave the whole job until they could give him an anaesthetic. His ankle was shattered. All hands were brought in to reduce the agony of the transference onto the bed. Nurse Sinclair winced as we lifted him.

A buzzer in Ward Two was going like a demented bee. Dashing in to deal with the emergency, I found a yelling Mr Harper. He had asked for a bedpan five minutes ago and hadn't got it yet. 'I'll get it myself,' he threatened with a grin.

'All right, all right,' I snapped, 'I'll get you one straight away. No need to make such a fuss.'

In the corridor Sister delayed me for a minute on my way to the sluice. My hand was reaching up to the bedpan rack when I heard a deafening crash, followed by screams and all the buzzers in Ward Two. Roger just beat me into the ward. Mr Harper's bed had toppled over and was lying askew, the top of the frame supported by the next bed. Mr Harper was hanging in mid-air, head down, body twisted and his whole weight on his broken leg; he was screaming. Roger had no choice; he cut the cords and we lowered him to the floor.

The ashen-faced patient on his right, mercifully out of bed at the time, told us that within a minute of my leaving the ward Mr Harper had announced: 'She's not coming—better go myself,' and promptly made one of his I'm-getting-up-if-you-don't-watch-out moves. As he did so the weights swung over and the foot of the bed slipped off the blocks, bringing the whole contraption crashing down.

When help arrived we righted the bed and put him back, lying flat. We were dumbfounded; no one had ever done anything like this before. He too was stunned. There was no doubt he had not intended this to happen; it had merely been a wild gesture. He was also in pain.

Mr Cartwright treated him to the full force of his fury and a chastened Mr Harper was conveyed to the theatre, where a pin was inserted below the knee so that more direct traction could be applied. It was more uncomfortable and hampering than the first arrangement but he didn't complain overmuch.

Boredom was the biggest problem with these healthy but immobile patients. Few seemed to have inner resources and there was little enthusiasm for occupational therapy. But they managed to be very interested in everything *we* did, which could be a bit wearing, especially with the long-termers who had picked up a bit of superficial knowledge, thereby becoming authorities, as men are wont to do.

The father of one of our younger ex-patients was 'in toys' and, three weeks before Christmas, sent us a big box of good quality assorted toys, all new but broken in some small way. We gave them to the patients to mend and suddenly they were happy and engrossed as never before. In the men's ward, toy trains straddled hip-plasters whilst couplings were repaired. Bed-tables became

44

test tracks for racing cars and pull-along toys, or served as operating tables when major orthopaedic surgery was performed on teddy bears and dolls. Peas were unbunged from whistles and numerous nurses gunned down the minute they were silhouetted in the ward doorway.

As it was a male ward, the element of competition entered into things. It became a point of honour to do the difficult repair oneself and not to hand it on to someone else. Even so, specialists did emerge in certain fields. Mr Harper, who was slowly and shamefacedly beginning to accept the confines of his position, proved to be a dab hand at railway engines.

It was going to be a lovely Christmas. It always was on Smithfield, they told me. The children got so utterly spoilt that some of last year's patients who were now quite well asked if they could come back in for Christmas. Aided by advice from all sides. we hung streamers and decorated the Christmas tree. I knew everyone and was becoming settled in.

But on 23rd December I was moved to another hospital in the group: the Shelley Infectious Diseases Hospital two miles away.

CHAPTER V

Stormy Nightingale

I leaned forward and firmly grasped the young man's neck and legs. Sister had emphasized the importance of keeping his spine well extended. The capped and gowned doctor had painted all the skin on Edward's lower back, surrounded it with sterile towels, and injected a local anaesthetic. Now he picked up the lumbar puncture needle and looked at me over his mask.

'Got him nice and firm, Nurse?'

I nodded.

'You will feel a slight prick, Edward,' he warned.

I took a deep breath and tried not to flinch as he inserted the needle between Edward's third and fourth lumbar vertebrae. When he was satisfied that it was deep enough he straightened for a moment, then bent again and removed the stylet. Nothing happened. Very cautiously he advanced the needle a fraction, and was rewarded with milky drops of cerebro-spinal fluid which gradually increased to a steady flow. Everyone relaxed, except me. The young doctor, clearly relieved at the success of this sometimes tricky operation, attached a glass tube to the needle and measured the pressure of the fluid. It was high. We were not surprised. Edward had been admitted as a suspected meningo-coccal meningitis and was very ill. We hadn't found any of the characteristic haemorrhagic spots which sometimes accompany this acute infectious disease, but the opaqueness of the fluid and its high pressure supported the meningitis diagnosis.

After taking specimens, the doctor withdrew the needle and sealed the puncture hole with a collodion dressing. I straightened up and massaged my back. Now we had to wait for the lab. report to name the cause of the meningitis. The initial symptoms were similar in all types, so lab. examination was required to tell us which organism was responsible. Only then could we start proper treatment. If it was the infectious and often lethal meningococcus, it could mean the start of an epidemic or it might just be an isolated case. If one of the other causal organisms such as streptococcus, pneumococcus, influenza, staphylococcus or T.B., it could still be serious but not liable to cause an epidemic.

Edward was glad to be left alone in a darkened room (his eyes were hyper-sensitive to light) with his pains and misery. He was extremely irritable, but this was a sympton of his disease.

A stint in Infectious Diseases was part of our general training and we supplemented the hospital's own staff who were mainly trainee Fever Nurses. I was on 'A' Ward which was mostly 'closed' chests. 'Closed' meant that, whilst some of the cases might be suffering from T.B., none were infectious. This was deduced by sputum examination; if the tubercular bacilli could be isolated, they were infectious and 'open'.

'A' was a pleasant, modern bungalow building standing on its own amid grassy lawns, as were all the wards at Shelley Infectious Diseases Hospital, or 'The Isolation' as it was known locally. We called it the I.D.

The ward was divided into single and double rooms. The two boys, aged twelve and thirteen, in Room Eight were would-be lechers. Both had suffered from attacks of pleurisy and, though now recovered, were being detained for several months as it was possible that T.B. was the underlying cause. They had a lot of enforced rest and were boyishly playful at first but, to our

47

surprise, they began to make saucy remarks and develop violent crushes. It was really a means of alleviating their boredom but some of the nurses were quite shocked and this of course made the boys worse. Peter, a quite handsome thirteen-year-old, developed a thing about me and his bell was always ringing when I was on duty. I was amused and a little flattered and as they were a light relief compared with some of the patients I was easy-going with them. Too easy-going, I was to discover.

One of the other doubles contained three 'broncho-babies'. The winter always brought an influx of babies suffering from broncho-pneumonia. Two were almost recovered and due for discharge, whilst a third was holding his own. Here I tried my hand at baby-feeding and nappy-changing though Nurse Sinclair, who had followed me over from St Margaret's, couldn't bear the sight and would groan and close her eyes at my awkwardness. She declared me the most unmaternal girl she'd ever met, which didn't bother me too much as I found babies a bit of a bore and couldn't understand why people enjoyed dandling and cooing at such semi-inanimate objects.

Jennifer, the five-month-old broncho-baby in Room Seven, was not responding to treatment. She had been deserted by her mother and no one ever came to see her. This distressed Nurse Sinclair very much. She was sure that if mother appeared the baby would miraculously improve, that it knew that no one cared. She spent any spare time sitting beside the oxygen tent, keeping the baby company. I couldn't see that it made any difference as I was sure the baby wouldn't know her mother if she saw her and wasn't capable of realizing anything. I tried to feel very upset about it, said lots of sympathetic things and looked sad like the others, but I was faking. Try as I would it seemed like an object rather than a person to me. Nurse Sinclair was unable to prove her theory as the baby died without mother reappearing.

Nurses went out with the ambulance that collected broncho-babies from their homes. Before setting out we were usually informed whether the baby was dangerously ill. I had no such warning on my first sortie, but the baby turned out to be critically ill and, as we pelted through the rush-hour traffic 'on the bell', I spent a harrowing time clasping a blue-faced, panting baby to my bosom, expecting my shaky artificial respiration to be put to the crucial test at any minute.

But on that occasion I was lucky, my skill remained untried and the baby was still breathing, albeit only just, when the ambulance swung through the hospital gates. But this experience did not help when, two babies later, I was sent out for a dangerously ill case.

'Take oxygen, an ampoule of coramine and a syringe,' said Sister. Coramine is used in trying to resuscitate the heart when it has stopped. 'Yes,' I said weakly, wondering who would die first, the baby or me.

It was a suitably dark, foggy night in the usual murky part of town (undernourishment is a pre-disposing factor in the disease), and we couldn't find the street. It was one of those ill-lit, ill-marked side turnings. We got out, peered at the street names until we found the right one and then had to wander round with lamps, looking for the number. Certainly no one was looking out for us. With my flowing cape and lamp held high, I must have looked like old Florrie herself doing her 'How are you soldier?' Crimea bit. But I was too worried to see the humour of the situation. When we finally found the right number, they took their time answering and looked surprised to see us.

'Didn't expect *you* so soon,' muttered the drab, carpet-slippered mum and added grudgingly: 'You better come in.'

The father and two children glanced briefly from their fish and chips as we entered. Mum's plateful was half eaten. There was no sign of baby.

'Where's the baby?' I asked.

'Oh, through there.' The woman nodded vaguely towards a closed door. 'You want a cup of tea?'

'No, thank you,' I answered a trifle touchily and made my way towards the other room.

'You're in a hurry!' she exclaimed as she led me through.

The baby lay sleeping peacefully, with a grubby dummy on her cheek. Breathing was a bit rapid, but she didn't look very ill to me. Seemed a pity to disturb her.

'Second time she's been in for it,' remarked the woman chattily, almost proudly.

I carried the baby out. Mum didn't bother to come to the door—her chips were getting cold.

At first, we were pleased when the lab. announced that Edward's meningitis was not meningococcal but tubercular. But we soon realized that it didn't make much difference to Edward. T.B. was widespread in his body and infecting other organs. His weight, poor on arrival, had dwindled rapidly and it was unpleasant to administer intra-muscular injections into his almost non-existent muscles, especially as it seemed so futile. His body did not respond and he was slipping away from us fast.

Everything about Edward had an air of deprivation and neglect. His ragged clothes and dirty skin on arrival, the meagre belongings on his locker, his coarse manner and his sparse visitors. He was a have-not and was always likely to be. What's more he was dying painfully. It outraged my sense of justice—it was not fair.

Whilst we were waiting for suppers to arrive, one of the buzzers sounded. It was Room Eight again. I took my time. Lately, Peter had been buzzing on any pretext. I would have to be firm with him; this crush business was going too far.

When I popped my head around the door, Peter said sweetly, 'May I have some more water, please, Nurse?'

Reasonable request, I thought and crossed to his locker for the jug.

'Oh, and my pillows, Nurse, I can't seem to get them right—could you?'

I leaned across and picked up a pillow. Peter looked up and shouted, 'Right!'

At this Harry jumped out of bed, closed the door and switched off the lights. At the same time Peter grabbed me, pulled me across the bed and kissed me! It all happened so suddenly and was so well organized that I was taken completely off guard—not that one expects patients to drag one onto the bed. When my brain started functioning again, I nearly died of panic. What if someone came in! Who would believe my innocence? I struggled like a beetle on its back. He had me at a disadvantage; I couldn't get purchase to push myself up from the bed and Harry was being a great help—to Peter.

'If you don't let me go, I'll scream this place down!' I spluttered furiously. 'I'll—I'll report you to Matron—to Dr Hawkins!' I had no intention of doing any such thing but the threat worked. Peter, who now seemed a bit disconcerted by his action, was not quite sure what to do next—he released me. I was furious and my fury, I'm told, can be intimidating. I unleashed it. Till now they had only seen a mild and easy-going me and were stunned.

'It was only a bit of fun, Nurse,' pleaded Peter weakly.

'Fun! Fun!' I yelled. 'My God—what if someone had come in—think of the trouble you could have caused me!'

It was obvious that such a thought had never crossed their minds. After that, I had more respect and no further trouble. Needless to say, I didn't report them to anyone: I knew who would have been blamed.

I had not realized that I would be capable of hating someone who was dying. It didn't happen like that in fiction—the heroine tends the suffering male with infinite kindness and patience and he is wan but grateful. But I hated Mr Phillipson and tended him as little as possible. He was dying of T.B., though it wasn't very obvious. True, he was thin and confined to bed but he did not appear very ill. I found this sentence of death on an apparently whole man dramatic and sad, at first. But Mr Phillipson was a b——. He treated the nurses like dirt, but in a superior, sardonic way, for he was a cultured man. He complained constantly, flew into rages and ordered us hither and thither.

No one stood up to him. Because he was dying and because his wife was a member of the staff, everyone had to be careful with Mr Phillipson, make sure he got his dinner first (and only the choicest portions), answer his bell at the double, fulfil his every curt demand, prevent his rages at all costs and, when they did occur, tolerate them. This of course made him progressively worse. He was like a small child seeing how far he could go and becoming desperate for a little spirited opposition. The staff were all very discontented but didn't *do* anything.

He saw straight away that my nature was not going to allow me to kowtow like the rest, however. But I had no wish to provoke trouble, so did my best to control my temper and keep out of his way. In any case, I knew I was no match for his quick and clever tongue. But he wanted the total submission of all and decided to break me. He goaded me at every opportunity. When I was about to perform a service for him he would curtly order me to do it so that I had to obey or stop what I was doing, which was usually impractical. I trained myself not to answer him and this spurred him on to greater efforts. Eventually I spoke to Sister, telling her that I was not going to be treated like a peasant by that ignorant balding autocrat. He would be better if *someone* was firm with him. She entreated me to be patient 'for his wife's sake'. She said she would speak to him. She did. He was worse after that and made jibes suggesting that his position was quite inviolable, he could do what he liked and I might just as well accept the fact.

The showdown came one evening when I went in to settle him down for the night. His 'settling down' had to be done at a precise time and all at once, not in the normal rounds that did for everyone else.

'Ah yes, Nurse Driscoll. Fill my water jug, wash the glass, take out my flowers, empty the bottle and draw the curtains—in that order,' he commanded.

He knew this was precisely what I had come in to do. I didn't say anything, but dealt with the water and the flowers.

'Empty my bottle now,' he ordered.

I made for the curtains.

'I told you to empty my bottle first and *then* draw the curtains!' he shouted.

Everything went black.

'Who the hell do you think you are?' I bellowed. 'Sitting there like a bloody sultan and ordering me about! You ignorant pig!'

I stormed out and found Sister while my fury was still raging. This time nothing would make me change my mind, I told her. I was going to Matron in the morning. Sister panicked and begged me to reconsider—for his wife's sake. I would refrain from going to Matron, only if I never, but never, had to go into his room again, I announced dramatically. To my amazement she agreed! She told the rest of the staff, who thought it a bit thick that they should have to put up with him all the time, but nonetheless were rather pleased at the gesture.

Sister went out of her way to keep her word and as there were plenty of staff it worked and I never entered his room again while I was on the ward. The other staff informed me that Mr Phillipson was a little subdued for a while and puzzled by my absence. Eventually, when he discovered the truth, he made remarks like,

53

'I understand that Nurse Driscoll is frightened to come in here', knowing that they would be repeated to me.

It mustn't be supposed that I was always brave in the face of authority. On the contrary, I was a bit of a coward and would accept too much abuse. But I had an over-developed sense of fair play and a temper which, when roused, swept away all caution, fear of retribution, fear of authority, anxiety over job, everything. Not control, though—never was I more icily controlled and lucid. When I calmed down I would think, Oh Gawd—what have I stirred up now? Tales about my digging-in of heels soon earned me an undeserved reputation for not giving a damn, which was a joke—I gave lots of damns.

A wonder drug which appeared to have magical, curative qualities in many diseases had been developed but no one was sure how wide were its potential uses or how lasting its effects. The doctors decided to try it on Edward. One thing was certain, it could not make the prognosis worse; there was no doubt he was dying. The effect was dramatic and almost immediate. His headaches and sensitivity to light were alleviated and he began to emerge from his cabbage-like existence and take an interest in the world around him.

Within a couple of weeks he was putting on weight and his complexion was losing some of its greyness. Vile temper gave way to cheek and a touch of arrogance, brought on partly by being the centre of attention for once in his life. He wasn't very likeable; deprivation doesn't make 'nice' people and that bit about suffering being good for one's soul is a lot of codswallop. But we were genuinely delighted, watched avidly and reported each sign of improvement. We felt he had cheated death and might have his chance after all. It was a miracle.

. . . . .

While we were straightening Peter's bed he kept fidgeting and glancing at me, as if trying to make up his mind about something. Eventually, he could contain himself no longer. He cleared his throat.

'Hey, Nurse Driscoll, you know that girl I've been waving to over on the T.B. block?'

'Yes,' I answered.

The waving took place when the beds were put out on the terraces. T.B. patients have a reputation for being sex-obsessed, but again I think this may be caused by long periods of boring confinement rather than being any manifestation of the disease. Our patients often carried on long-distance intrigues amongst themselves—or fell violently for the nurses. No one took much notice, for it kept them happy.

We had passed on childish verbal messages from the boys to this girl and back. Her nurses were sorry for her as she was younger than the rest of the patients, and lonely.

'Well,' said Peter, 'I wrote to her and I just got a reply. Look.' With a touch of bravado, he thrust the letter into my hand. 'What do you think of that?'

'Dear Peter,' I read aloud for the benefit of my colleague, 'Thank you very much for your letter. . . .' Mundane platitudes followed which I gabbled swiftly—we had to finish the beds. 'Yes,' I went on, 'I would like to meet you when we leave hospital. I bet you are very handsome.' Peter was watching my face intently now. 'We could go for a walk in the spinney and you could kiss me and then you could take my knickers off and lay on top of me and . . .' My voice trailed away into astonished silence. The boys sniggered and blushed.

'Good God!' I exclaimed. 'Who *is* this girl? I've never read anything like that in my life! What on earth did you write to get an answer like that?'

'Nothing, Nurse Driscoll, honest. Just ordinary things—ask

55

Harry. I don't know anything about her 'cept she's fifteen and a half.'

He was obviously disconcerted by the depths of passion into which his latest sortie into the grown-up world of sex had landed him. Though he would never have admitted it, he was clearly shocked.

'You're definitely not to write back and I'm going to tell the other nurses to stop this passing of messages,' I insisted.

'Aw,' groaned Harry, 'Spoil-sport,' and glared at Peter.

But Peter, though he made protesting noises, was obviously relieved at my insistence.

Dragging a nurse onto the bed and kissing her—well, that was different, a bit of fun—but this was beyond a joke.

I spent most of my first stint of nights on Ward 'D' and some of my more outstanding memories are: a couple of horribly deformed spinal bifidas, one of them having the huge head of the hydrocephalic (water on the brain), waiting to die; my first experience of nursing a patient in an iron lung (a bad polio epidemic was just starting); my low physical ebb around 4 a.m.; the night-duty taste in my mouth at breakfast; and the surprise that I was suddenly thought capable of dealing with any emergency or nursing procedure. But most of all, I remember my few nights in solitary charge of 'F' Ward.

'F' Ward, housed in an old building, had only a handful of patients in one bare, high-ceilinged room and they were all young children. I spent most of the night in the modernized kitchen which from waist-height on the outside wall was all window. None of the other wards was visible, only a sea of blackness fringed by shadowy bushes and trees.

There were frequent rumours of prowlers and it was certainly easy enough to get into the grounds. Once in, the isolation of the wards made it a haven for the would-be snooper. I felt very vulnerable.

I always arrived for duty determined that tonight I was not going to be frightened: it was all in my imagination. But after the day staff had left a hush fell, when I became aware of creaking sounds from the old woodwork and the trees rustling in the wind. I began to feel watched. A tempting ware exhibited in a brightly lit shop window for the customers out there in that inky blackness which my eyes could not penetrate, no matter how hard I tried. More creaks, rustlings and the odd, banging door would gradually make me more jumpy and I would work myself into a state of near hysteria. Sometimes I'd escape the exposed kitchen to stand in the ward beside the sleeping children. They were all far too young to be of any assistance in fending off the bogey man, but at least they were company.

One night I heard a rattle at the kitchen door and looked up to see a strange man, head down, his coat collar shielding his face. I aged ten years as he looked up, revealing himself as a young relief doctor making an unexpected call in the rain.

'You look as if you've seen a ghost, Nurse Sinclair,' he laughed. 'Why do you lock the door? Are you scared? We'll have to give you something for your nerves!'

All right for your bloody sex, I thought (not for the first time), but said a trifle petulantly, 'My name is Driscoll—*not* Sinclair!'

To be fair, although confessing to some nervousness, few of the other nurses who did this lone stint seemed to suffer as I did; most were of the rational 'Who would want to sneak around here and attack us?' line of thought, which gave me little comfort.

My only distraction was exercising my imagination in writing the night report in the large tome provided. Since the children were mostly asleep when I arrived at 8 p.m. and I had only seen them in a dim light since, I felt there was little I could say about them. But my predecessors seemed to have culled much information from their inert bodies.

My complete ignorance of fevers did not help (we had fever lectures in the third year), but I studied the previous night reports and gradually developed the requisite knack of saying nothing in several different ways. When there was absolutely nothing to report about their general condition, 'Good night', 'No change', 'Comfortable', and 'Slept well' filled the bill. Any slight deviation was seized upon gratefully. If a child woke up and asked for a glass of water one could put 'Restless night'. 'Complained of headache, aspirin, $2\frac{1}{2}$ grains, administered and relief obtained' was another proof that I hadn't slept all night. Comments on general conditions were interspersed with the seemingly obligatory note on the continuing saga of *the rash*—whether it was spreading, fading or desquamating (my *Nurses' Dictionary* informed me that this meant peeling) and where.

Although I lost track of many patients when moving about so much, the mealtime gossip kept me informed about those in which I was more interested. Before I returned to St Margaret's I learned that Edward was regressing as fast as he had improved on the wonder drug. So much for our miracle.

'You will help the porter to take the body to the mortuary; there's no one else available,' said Night Sister briskly.

At 3 a.m. the porter arrived and we set out with the trolley along the concrete paths which chopped up the grounds into neat symmetrical patches. The night was very dark and a fine drizzle was wilting my cap so I pulled up my hood, which crushed it instead. Damn, I'd just made it and it had to last several nights.

The mortuary was tucked away in a discreet corner near the main gates.

'You're not scared, are you?' leered the tall, dark, saturnine porter.

'Of course not!' I laughed casually. 'I've seen plenty of dead people—a few more won't make any difference.'

I certainly wasn't scared of bodies, especially the one we had with us; I'd known the one-time occupant. But I *was* scared of the dark.

I began to feel a bit creepy as we neared the small brick building nestling amongst the dense bushes and the tall trees which moved in the wind. It was the living who worried me; I was convinced they hid behind every bush, awaiting the opportunity to attack.

'They say it's haunted,' whispered the porter confidentially.

'That's very original of them,' I retorted sarcastically, as he made much of creeping off to unlock the double doors.

Nevertheless I pushed the trolley as far as it would go up to the edge of the ramp, while attempting to look behind me and keep my eye on him simultaneously. He took his time unlocking, then popped inside to unbolt the other door.

Suddenly I heard a strangled cry! The porter staggered out backwards round the door—there were hands around his neck! The strangled sounds came from his throat as he struggled. I screamed in sheer terror.

'Here, take it easy!' he said, turning round to reveal that they were his own hands. 'You'll have the whole bloody hospital here. What a noise—enough to wake the dead!' He thought that was hilarious.

Once inside with the lights on, they were just a lot of bodies covered with sheets. Bodies of people whom you have never known in life are odd: just lumps of nothing. I tried to imagine them animated but it did not work.

'Come and look at this one,' said the porter chattily. 'Doesn't she look nice?'

He pulled back the sheet to reveal a dark-haired, gentle-faced woman in her mid-twenties. Her cheeks retained a slight rosy glow.

'Keep their colour with gas poisoning. Makes them look much better, doesn't it?' he suggested, with professional interest.

'Suicide?' I asked.

'Yes, her old man was carrying on with someone else. She went to the fish and chip shop, got six bob changed into shillings and then put her head in the gas oven. Shame. She looks nice.'

I agreed it seemed a terrible waste.

CHAPTER VI

Tempestuous Nightingale

'The diagnosis isn't made here until the post mortem,' said the third-year nurse cynically. 'Here' was Maxwell, the medical ward. I had pestered her to tell me what four consecutive patients were suffering from and each time she had replied that they were query such and such and so and so or they were in for investigations. A few nurses liked all this mystery and deduction, but I found it irritating and much preferred the straightforward 'look, see and cut it out' of surgical.

Of course, many patients *were* diagnosed and the majority were suffering from, to use their own words, cardiac hearts, gastric stomachs, ulsters, and too much sugar in the blood, Nurse, though I've never had a sweet tooth. I think the vagueness of it all irritated the patients as well, for they were a grumpy lot. The fact that most gastrics are worrying types and the hearts rather naturally frightened and self-obsessed certainly contributed to this and the irksome restrictions on diet and habits did not help.

On night duty at the I.D., I had been expected to be quite responsible but now, once again, I was reduced to being the unreliable novice. As there was not a great deal of special work for seniors on the ward, anything requiring the slightest degree of skill went to them. It was the sluice, wiping, flowers, meals and bedpans again for me. I was allowed a couple of skilled jobs, though the honour was a doubtful one: testing endless diabetic urines and collecting specimens of faeces in jolly little bottles with toy spoons in the lid.

When emptying bedpans and bottles we were always required to 'observe the contents' (quantity, colour, consistency, odour and abnormal contents), but it was especially important on medical. There were several poetic stock descriptions to guide me. Abnormal stools could be anything from frothy to pea-soup and abnormal urine could smell fishy or of new-mown hay. Normal urine was 'straw-coloured or resembling sherry' ('That's a fine Amontillado you've got there!' 'Oh no, more of a Fino, I'd say'!).

These exercises came under the heading of 'Observation of vomit, sputum, urine and stools'. It was the second of this well-known comedy team that I could not stomach. I could quite happily test oceans of urine and even got used to the pong (or characteristic odour as it was officially termed) of faeces, but emptying sputum mugs made me heave. Nowadays they are disposable but our metal mugs had to be emptied and cleaned.

I would invert the mug over the sluice flush pan then turn my head away and hope that gravity, never my friend, would do its bit. Too often it didn't and I would turn around to see one long yellow glutinous lump suspended between mug and basin, waiting to be released. Sputum was my Waterloo. I'm afraid not much of it was closely observed by me.

While all of this was going on after breakfast, another of the juniors was getting the flowers out after their night's sojourn in the sluice, change of water and removal of the dead. En route she would have to suffer, 'I didn't get my chrysanths at all yesterday,' (instead of telling us yesterday, the patients would rather wait until today and really feel martyrs), or the indignant 'What's happened to all my dahlias?', as if we had stolen some of the slimy, dead things to decorate the bedpan washer. If we were lucky one of the patients took over this chore.

.   .   .   .   .

Other memories of the medical ward are fragmentary. I remember when we had to crawl around on our knees to make the bed of an epileptic woman who was being nursed on the floor because we could no longer restrain her in a bed. A skeletal, prematurely old woman, she had many scars from falls and burns sustained during attacks. She had begun to deteriorate mentally and would do anything to gain our attention, even staging mock epileptic fits to this end. We had put her in a single room because of her disturbing effect on other patients and it soon became obvious that a normal bed was of no use; she kept hurling herself floorwards. We tried a high-sided cot, but she insisted on climbing onto the edge and perching there like a vulture until one of us opened the door, when she would dramatically launch herself into the air. We couldn't stand the strain. Various devices to keep her in, without totally immobilizing her, were merely a challenge to her ingenuity.

Eventually, we capitulated and put her mattress on the floor. It was interesting to see doctors and the immensely tall consultant physician trying to retain their aplomb when on their knees examining her.

Meal times were trying for both patients and staff. The deprivation or cosseting of individuals with special diets (low fat, high protein, low salt, diabetic, etc.) engendered self-pity in some and guilt in others. The diabetics were often admitted for the purpose of stabilization: that is, to achieve the right balance, for them, of food and insulin. By the time we'd messed about weighing bits of potato and such, the food was invariably cold and unappetizing.

I remember the time I grabbed a cup from the sink and quaffed my fill of water, when dying of thirst after the pre-visiting time rush. George, one of the male nurses, laughed evilly when he saw what I'd done.

'They'll never believe that's how you got it,' he said, slowly turning the cup around until I saw the tell-tale mark on the side.

It was Mr McBride's special crockery and Mr McBride was a W.R. positive.

'What a shame,' said George sympathetically, 'getting syphilis in such a dull way after keeping yourself pure all this time.' He grinned hopefully. 'Might as well start enjoying yourself now!'

I always had difficulty remembering patients' names and diagnoses, which made the serving of special diets a nightmare. I would dash out with a tray, chanting to myself, 'from left to right—Mr Barker's diabetic, Mr Davidson's salt-free and Mr Muir's diabetic'. Then someone would ask me for a bottle or tell me the good news that they were going home, and I would have difficulty finding Mr Barker and when I did I would have forgotten which dinner was which and have to go back and ask Staff who would be furious and say I ought to know the patients by now. Because of this, Matron's phenomenal memory for the names, faces and diagnoses of all the people she saw so briefly on her rounds never failed to astound me.

One day I received a bouquet of crimson roses from Bill. They were to wish me luck for my 'first-part prelim'. The senior staff were astonished; they could not imagine how anyone as unimpressive as a first-year nurse could inspire such a gesture, much less acquire a boy-friend inclined to these extravagances. The bouquet was addressed to *Miss* Driscoll (Staff) and was taken to the sisters' dining-room first, as a matter of course!

There were continuous complaints about the strength of the tea and the consistency of the morning eggs. Tea was a seemingly insoluble problem on all wards. Tastes vary so and one could never satisfy everyone. The same pot could provoke cries of

'What a lovely cup of tea, Nurse!'

or

'You call this *tea*?'

'Too weak!'

'Too strong!'

One cardiac was always announcing that Nurse Driscoll was the only one who knew how to make a good cup of tea, merely because I made it weak, the way he liked it. Most of the other men groaned when I poured 'that wee-wee again', but it was quite popular in the women's ward.

The morning eggs were something else. Many of the patients preferred boiled eggs to any of the other breakfast dishes offered ('that muck') and the gastrics in particular needed soft-boiled eggs. There were so many (mostly the patients' own 'fresh' eggs of varying ages) that it was impossible to boil them individually, so they were done in one large pan, which made correct timing difficult. The usual complaint was 'too hard'.

One group of well-known male dissidents became neurotic about the subject and I determined to achieve success if only to thwart them. I made a supreme effort and divided the eggs into four and numbered them as I put them in, so that I could take them out in the same order. This must be *it*, I thought, as I raced around serving them before they had time to set. I waited timidly for the male verdict—the women had said that theirs were fine. The prime grumbler dismissed his with elaborate disgust, '*Raw!*' and pontificated, 'You can't have left them in long enough—I told you five minutes for mine!'

'Raw,' echoed his crony with eager satisfaction.

'Too hard,' said another. 'I don't know why you can't time an egg, it's simple enough!' Then the final straw.

'You've put it in the egg-cup upside down,' chipped in a bed-bound sultan.

That did it. I went pink to the ears and exploded.

'You make me sick, the lot of you!' I stood in the middle of the ward and shouted. 'You are worse than a lot of old women— nothing but grumble, grumble, grumble. I've never nursed such a lot of selfish old miseries. You ought to have babies. *That* would give you something to complain about!' (I had been hearing some gruesome tales from unfortunate colleagues who were being used as slave labour on the maternity wing.)

The effect was startling. Spoons froze 'twixt egg and mouth and yolk dripped onto slack chins. All chatter and animation were suspended as, wide-eyed, they watched me stalk off, emanating waves of fury and disgust. My Gala Performance was the talk of the ward for the rest of the day and relieved their boredom no end. They were fascinated by this new phenomenon and kept sneaking wondering looks at my once-again demure face. Tentative remarks such as, 'Here, we have got a temper, haven't we?' or, 'Some of them *do* drive you mad—always complaining!' were whispered conspiratorially in my ear. All were anxious to disassociate themselves from the 'selfish old miseries'!

I surpassed myself once by breaking a jar full of thermometers (six). We broke thermometers on purpose, in Matron's opinion anyway. That thermometers are fragile and a fair percentage of breakages are inevitable may seem obvious to you, but not to Matron. Whenever we broke one we had to pay a visit to her office at 9 a.m., wearing a clean cap and apron and clutching the remnants of the offending object. We were required to inform Matron how we broke it and suffer a berating if the explanation was considered unsuitable.

'I dropped it', 'It slipped out of my fingers when I was shaking it down', or 'A patient let it slip out of his mouth' were the obvious, and usually true, reasons but were considered *passé*.

So, like one's reasons for being late for work, they became the object of furious mental exercise and the resulting fiction more and more wildly improbable.

I became quite overwrought, thinking how inadequate 'I dropped them' seemed for six, but couldn't think how else I could explain it. 'I hurled them at the wall' hinted of deliberate intent. The jar had been broken as well, but that was just an old fish-paste jar with sticking plaster sectioning the mouth. Fish-paste jars were expendable and I could have used a mile of plaster for any purpose I desired, at least until the Assistant Matron's next *adhesive - plaster - must - not - be - used - for - labels* purge. But thermometers!

Mrs Cream Biscuits. Her real name was Riddle and she had been on the ward for some time. Originally admitted for some fairly minor bladder trouble shortly after the birth of her first baby, she had not responded to treatment and was being investigated further. She missed her baby terribly and had only glimpsed him twice since her admittance, but she was wonderfully cheerful and a great friend of mine. We were brought together by our common passion for custard creams. When she discovered our mutual addiction, she elected to keep me supplied and would inform me surreptitiously when a fresh batch arrived.

The awful day of the second part of the 'second-part prelim' examination—the practical. I had stayed at home the night before, travelled to the hospital with my mother and was due to enter the torture chamber at 9.30 a.m. I made my way to the P.T.S. where the practical was to be held, getting myself all worked up en route with violent attacks of pre-exam nerves. As the deadline approached, I suddenly realized that I had left my entrance pass in my mother's bag. The first onrush of panic subsided when I remembered that she was attending a lecture in the P.T.S. that morning. I did the last fifty yards to the building in record time and panted out my predicament ro the tutor in charge.

His answer was typical. Mrs Oppenheimer, the gynaecologist, was lecturing. Mrs Oppenheimer did not like to be interrupted. Quite out of the question to disturb Mrs Oppenheimer. When Mrs Oppenheimer finished at ten, I could get my card. But we would see if the examining sister would consider putting back my practical for half an hour.

I rushed down the corridor to the examination room where, after much pleading, the frosty-faced examiner reluctantly agreed. As ten drew nearer, the tutor and I waited outside the lecture-room. It seemed an age but at last ten o'clock came—and went. I was a mass of jelly by now and begged the tutor to interrupt. But no. This was most unusual of Mrs Oppenheimer, Mrs Oppenheimer nearly always finished on time, he couldn't remember the last time Mrs Oppenheimer had overrun. Mrs Oppenheimer was sure to finish any moment now. At seven minutes past ten the lecture ended. I tore in, saw Mum, grabbed my card, tore out and raced back to the examination room.

'No,' said the examiner, without a trace of regret in her voice, 'you are too late.'

I can't remember what I said to the tutor when it sunk in that I would have to sit the whole thing—both parts—again in three months' time *and* pay the fee (half a week's wage). I *can* remember that when I returned to the hospital (still pristine in my specially made cap and spotless apron) and was surrounded by colleagues asking,

'What was it like?'

'Who was your examiner?'

'What bed did you get?'

and someone handed me Bill's now traditional bunch of red roses, I burst into tears.

But that wasn't quite the end of the matter. I had also, of

course, to attend Matron's office for my official dressing down for 'failing to sit my exam'.

I was on theatre again. It was going to be a nice, quiet evening. The list had been short and everything was cleared up by the time I returned from my afternoon off. Unless there was a sudden emergency, Nurse Peebles and I could have a peaceful chat over a gauze-folding and glove-patching session, and I could get off on time to meet Bill. Nurse Peebles chatted, in desultory fashion, about the afternoon list. It was finished even earlier than anticipated, despite Mr Prentiss's pedantic fiddling about, because the possible big abdominal had turned out to be inoperable and had been closed up again after only a brief look.

'Simply chocker with carc.,[1]' commented Nurse Peebles sadly, 'and only a young woman too.'

Again I tutted and made sympathetic noises but felt uneasy. I didn't really feel very much about it. I was beginning to suspect that I must be terribly hard; death and suffering didn't seem to touch me as much as it should.

The quiet in the isolated, empty theatre suite was uncanny and the clean orderliness surrounding us increased the atmosphere of peaceful retreat. Remnants of a pale sun filtered through the window and glinted on the instrument cupboard and huge chrome-topped cauterizing machine. We nestled into our cosy gossip as our hands mechanically snipped and folded, stuck and patched. What a lovely evening. Even Sister seemed to have forgotten her threat to ask us the names and functions of all the surgical instruments.

The rude interruption came at 7.20 p.m. when Nurse Peebles was at supper. Sister popped her head round the door.

'There's a panic on Fieldman. Go up there and help them get ready for visiting.'

[1] Carcinoma, a type of cancer.

I groaned. When wasn't there a panic on Fieldman? To be dragged away from my reverie was bad enough, but then to be thrown into that insane maelstrom was too much, my nerves wouldn't stand it.

Fieldman, the surgical ward, had op. lists daily and was on admittance permanently. There was nowhere else to send emergencies. A nearby hospital had a surgical ward but no major theatre, so they mostly got Fieldman's semi-convalescents. The number of patients requiring intensive care at any one time on Fieldman was incredible.

I brightened en route. A lively break might be welcome after all; the edge-of-hysteria atmosphere was bracing, to say the least, but bearable when one was not personally responsible for having everything cleared up for the night staff. Anyway one was inclined to become unsociable on theatre and patients were always so nice to visiting nurses who didn't know their nasty habits.

As I passed the growing queue of visitors outside Fieldman, a shy young man, grasping a bunch of drooping anemones, stepped forward and touched my arm.

'Hello, Nurse Driscoll. It's a long time since we've seen you. My wife has missed you.'

It was Mr Riddle, alias Mr Cream Biscuits. I was delighted but puzzled.

'Why are you in this queue? Your wife's on Maxwell.'

He grinned. 'Not now she isn't. They finally decided to operate and find out what's wrong. I'm to see the doctor when I go in. It'll be nice to know where we are.' He smiled hopefully.

'Must dash—see you later, perhaps—I'm giving them a hand in there.'

'Give her my love if she's round. She'll be pleased to see you,' he called after me.

One did miss personal contact, I mused, as I knocked on Sister's door.

'You'd better ask Nurse Dawson what she would like you to do,' said Sister.

I managed to convey this query to Nurse Dawson as she flashed between ward and sluice. Her body was having a little trouble keeping up with her feet. Nurses on Fieldman never stopped moving to speak and I got my answer as she whipped out of the sluice and into the medicine room. It sounded like 'elp urs oates eds into'. But I had acquired one useful skill in the theatre—de-garbling. I could de-garble the most obscure message, as long as I had an idea of what the original intent might be and could work back from there. This was obviously 'Help Nurse Coates with the beds in Two'. But a frantic Nurse Coates was just wheeling the bed trolley out of Two and I followed her into Three, the women's ward.

'Come on, Nurse, our visitors will be late in again!' exclaimed a pinkly-plump woman done up like the bon-bon she wasn't in a pink lacy bedjacket with satin bows.

'I'm going as fast as I can,' wailed Coatsie. 'Don't worry, we'll let them stay overtime.'

'Make sure you tell that to the night staff!' grumbled a hatchet-faced woman with a pinched little mouth. I bet someone was dying to see her!

A cosy purple dressing-gown topped by an anxious but kind face trotted up, 'I've tidied all the locker-tops and got rid of any bedpans,' she assured us. 'Mrs Oliver's is on the side in the sluice with her name on.'

Ah, the ward mother.

'Bless you, dear,' said Nurse Coates. 'Don't know what I'd do without you.'

'I think they make you girls work far too hard,' said pink bon-bon as we left her and started on the next bed.

'Oh, Nurse,' she called me back, 'could you just pour me a glass of water and hand me my handkerchief from the other side of the locker? Sorry to bother you—pulls my stitches if I struggle to do it myself.' She looked down affectionately at her pink satin abdomen.

'I bet,' muttered Nurse Coates under her breath.

The gaunt but smiling woman in the next bed smoothed her top sheet and whispered: 'It's all right, my dear, I've straightened, it up. Don't waste time on me.'

As we dashed gratefully on Coatsie asked over her shoulder, 'How are you feeling now? You weren't too bright this afternoon, were you?'

'I'm fine, fine. Isn't this the young lady I had a chat with when I went to theatre?'

'Yes, that's right,' I smiled. I thought the face was familiar. Oh, I remembered now—the nephrectomy where the water-logged kidney turned out to be so huge.

'Needn't bother with this one either,' said my colleague, automatically looking up to check the blood in the drip bottle. 'She's not long back from theatre and she's hardly moved. Pity she's got to come round at all, poor dear. She's inoperable— abdominal carc.'

Oh, this was her. Out of mildly morbid curiosity I moved to the top of the bed for a closer look at her still face. It was familiar.

'Oh, no!'

'What's the matter?' asked Coatsie. 'You look shattered. Know her?'

'It's Mrs Cream Biscuits,' I stammered foolishly.

'Funny name—nickname?' she murmured absently and started on the next bed. 'Come on—don't just stand there looking at her. There's work to do.'

'Nurse,' whined the bon-bon, 'you forgot to push up my bed-table.' She was struggling gamely to reach it, but managing to not quite make it. 'I hate to bother you, dear.'

'So you said,' I snapped tartly.

The visitors swarmed into the ward at 7.45 p.m., a quarter of an hour late. I waited in the kitchen, so as to avoid bumping into Mr Riddle, but as I left the ward he was still standing hesitantly at Sister's door, right hand raised to knock again and left hand grasping the anemones even more tightly as he listened. He brightened when he saw me.

'Did you——?'

'Come in,' interrupted Dr Barry's voice, to my great relief.

I nodded, forced a slight smile and fled.

CHAPTER VII

Fieldman—No Time to Stand and Stare

Mr Slack had fat ear-lobes, that was a help. I squeezed the right one, picked up my scalpel blade and made a tiny incision. Lovely rich blobs of scarlet sprang out and I caught them in my little bottle.

I shouldn't have been using a blade at all so I promptly hid it under a lump of cotton wool in the kidney dish. Large suture needles were the official instruments, but on the two occasions that I had tried them my poor victims had ended up with a lobe full of holes, made even more painful by the endless squeezing required to make them fruitful. Whilst I had got in a state, trying not to hurt but at the same time trying to obtain a specimen before the next one was due and thus avoid Staff's wrath at my slowness. After that I'd become a confirmed scalpel girl: a good primary cut to be re-opened every half hour.

That was enough. A piece of cotton wool on the ear and a label on the bottle. I handed Mr Slack a urine bottle, 'Right, do your duty.'

'The final indignity,' he sighed. 'Making water to order.'

He addressed himself to Mr Wartski, the Polish seaman in the next bed, who nodded and smiled in reply. Mr Wartski always nodded and smiled, for he understood not a word of English (apart from 'Good morning' which he used most indiscriminately). This hadn't made his treatment any easier; English hospitals are not normally overrun with Polish speakers.

When he was admitted, it had been obvious what was wrong: perforated peptic ulcer—the agonizing symptoms are fairly classic. He had been very ill after the emergency op. and while we fought for his life he had nodded and smiled very weakly. Now, something of a ward pet, he was giving us some concern for, just as he appeared to be recovering nicely, he seemed to be getting a chest infection which he was in no condition to fight. But he still nodded and smiled and said 'Good morning' at any time of the day or night.

Sometimes I wished it could be like a cinema hospital where the surgeon, peeling off his gloves, announces quietly but dramatically, 'The operation was a success. Jimmy will live.' Obviously, they had the edge on us—some secret drug which obviated any chance of complications.

'Drink this, please,' I requested.

Mr Slack took a mouthful and made an awful face, 'It's so sweet!'

'That's not surprising since it's glucose. Come on, you're worse than a child!'

He downed the rest with much fuss, deliberately guying it for Mr Wartski's amusement. I checked the time.

'Right, I'll be back at ten-thirty for more blood, eleven for blood and urine, eleven-thirty, blood, twelve, blood and urine.'

'Romantic assignments with a young maiden,' he sighed.

I'd better do that two-hourly aspiration. It had been due at ten and it was now ten past. I attached a large syringe to Mr Lowrie's nasal tube and drew back the plunger. The barrel filled with gastric juices—a nasty, brownish-green fluid. I expelled this into a container and repeated the exercise several times.

'They're leaving that tube in a long time,' commented the next patient. 'Mine was taken out a lot quicker.'

'Each case is different, Mr Lumley,' I admonished, mentally adding, and yours is more different than most.

'I was very ill!' he declared defensively.

'You certainly were,' I agreed, 'but as I said you can't generalize, these things vary.'

Like most nurses, I no longer noticed what a lying hypocrite I had become—it was so much part of the job.

Mr Lumley *had* been very ill when admitted. A gastric history and then those so characteristic signs and painful symptoms of a 'perf.'. He had undergone the typical emergency operation in the dead of night. But the mystified surgeon had found nothing amiss whatsoever, no matter how hard he looked. Nonetheless, the life-saving op. did the trick and Mr Lumley was losing the typical gaunt gastric face and worried expression. He was filling out, thriving, recovering like mad in fact and blessed the day he'd had his much-needed op. We could only presume he'd read some good books on the subject.

I checked Mr Lowrie's intravenous dextrose and saline drip for the umpteenth time. Nurses on Fieldman were compulsive drip-watchers and did an automatic 'eyes up' as they passed them, without breaking step or interrupting speech. We even got the patients at it and they would call behind the screens to us 'Mr Vincent's drip is getting low, Nurse' or 'The damn thing's stopped again, Nurse!'

This one was at the irritating phase when it was fairly low but not low enough to change the bottle over. It seemed to have been at the same level for ages, though when I checked the drip chamber it was dripping away steadily at the required forty-a-minute. I knew that as soon as I turned my back it would race like mad and try to empty before I could catch it. I'd better get a replacement out of the fridge so that it would be ready and warmed up.

'May I have a bottle, please?' asked Mr Lowrie, as I took his gastric juices towards the sluice to be measured.

'Me too, while you're there.'

That was the trouble with doing jobs in the ward: these blasted diversions for bottles, bedpans and glasses of water. Although Male Nurse James was in here as well, he was doing the dressings and was safe behind his important-looking mask and gown. Not that many patients asked him to get things anyway as he was third-year and not very obliging.

After I'd measured the brown fluid I knocked on Sister's door.

'Still four-point-three dextrose and eighteen per cent saline for Mr Lowrie, Sister?'

'Yes, Nurse. Wait a minute. You can give Mr Hetherington his pre-med.'

'Yes, Sister,' I groaned mentally. That's what I liked about this ward, one always got a chance to finish one job before——

I followed Sister's calm and impeccable figure to the medicine room. She was so clean, starched, spruce and serene that one wanted to touch her to see if she was real.

'One-third of a grain of omnopon and one-hundred-and-fiftieth of scopolamine. Check, Nurse.'

'One-third of a grain of omnopon and one-hundred-and-fiftieth of scopolamine. Check, Sister.'

'What does it do, Nurse?' she asked.

'What, Sister?' I asked, puzzled. My mind was busy: Mr Lowrie's aspiration, ten ounces to be charted, dextrose and saline for his drip and Christ it's ten-thirty, time for the second blood and I haven't done that other aspiration yet—was that all?

'Om. and scop., Nurse! You're not concentrating. What action does it have?'

Oh, I knew this one; we'd used it at the E.N.T. 'Omnopon is a hypnotic and scopolamine inhibits bronchial secretions, which makes it useful before general anaesthetics,' I parroted smugly. Being two of my first drugs and having funny names, they had stuck.

'Very good, Nurse. Give it immediately. It's ten-thirty-three.'

She marked his notes accordingly.

'Where's my bottle, Nurse?' asked Mr Lowrie and Co. in unison as I entered the ward with the syringe.

'I haven't forgotten, be patient.'

'That's all very well, Nurse; I hope you'll change the sheets.'

Pre-med. given, I dashed out again, got the dextrose and saline and grabbed two bottles on my way back.

'*That*'s not very hygienic, Nurse. Carrying intravenous fluid and urine bottles at the same time,' commented Staff severely. She always managed to make it sound as though I had some ghastly ulterior motive for such misdeeds, instead of being a victim of circumstance.

I changed the drip bottle, noted the ten ounces of aspiration and the litre of dextrose and saline on the Intake and Output chart, washed my hands and dashed over to Mr Slack. Thank goodness the cut opened again. Must get that second aspiration started.

I had half the sample when the doors flew open to admit a trolley, attended by the begowned porter and a nurse steadying a bottle of blood. It was the first of the morning's list back already.

'All hands!' yelled the porter. 'Everyone lazing about and disorganized, as usual!'

'Here,' I shoved the sample bottle into Mr Slack's hand, 'put the lid on and stick some wool on your ear.'

'Not moving till we get another one,' announced the porter arbitrarily.

Fortunately Nurse Foxley had seen the trolley enter and was following them in.

'Right. You here,' indicated the porter busily, 'and you at the top. Now lift. Careful.'

When he had extracted the lifting poles we automatically rolled the patient over to one side, pushing the canvas stretcher-cover under him, and then back again the other way to extract it completely, to the accompanying 'Roll him over' and 'Now back' from the porter.

I got Mr Slack's cut going again but it was more difficult this time. Nurse James came from behind the adjacent bed's screens and leered at me over his mask. When he was out of earshot, Mr Slack looked serious and rather embarrassed.

'He's got his eye on you, Nurse Driscoll.'

'How do you know?' I laughed.

'He told us, didn't he, Jack?' He addressed his mate behind the screens who peeped round and nodded vigorously. Mr Slack, Jack and the man in the next bed were all dears and had adopted me. They were cheerful, uncomplaining and very helpful.

'Well,' said Jack, 'we thought we'd better warn you. He's not really the sort of bloke you should get mixed up with,' he hinted darkly.

Mr Slack agreed. 'We don't think his intentions are honourable!'

I nearly hooted with laughter but they were so obviously doing their fatherly duty by me that I couldn't hurt their feelings.

'Don't worry,' I said, 'I've got a regular boy-friend and I'm not likely to fall for Mr James, no matter how attractive he is.'

'Oh, good, I told Jack you wouldn't be interested in him.'

I dashed out with the urine bottles and measured Mr Lowrie's. At last I started Mr Spencer's aspiration. He was yesterday's partial gastrectomy and still very ill.

Nurse Foxley, arms piled with linen, sped by.

'You've got to help me make up a bed—obstruction being admitted,' she threw at me as she started stripping Mr Rose's bed while he was still scrambling out of it. As an absent afterthought she asked, 'You *are* going home this afternoon, aren't you?'

He nodded and laughed.

I looked pleading. 'Oh Margaret, I can't I've——'

'Don't worry, I'll help Nurse Foxley,' Mr Rose assured me.

'Driscoll's slacking again, I see. *It won't do, Nurse!*' Foxley admonished, imitating a certain Staff Nurse's frozen tones.

I mouthed a familiar swear word at her. She always looked so serious and efficient the patients thought butter wouldn't melt in her mouth; it was hard to believe she was the same Nurse Foxley who had led us into scrapes at Penhurst.

In a moment of madness I had told her about this marvellous hospital and she had followed me a few months later. Tee-hee— she was junior to me on Fieldman. But in reality, any friends and classmates clung together; we could console one another and ask questions without either getting our heads bitten off, or fearing the results of the exposure of our ignorance, or both.

Mr Prentiss with his entourage of houseman, Sister and nurse had just entered the ward. I put the spigot back in Mr Spencer's nasal tube, did an eyes up at his drip and—damn, it had stopped!

Mr Prentiss reached the next bed to Mr Lowrie who was also one of his. He was bound to peruse the Intake and Output chart; he was fanatical about them. Still, that was all right, I'd entered the aspiration and intravenous solution—Oh Lor, I'd forgotten the urine!

I sauntered quietly over, hoping that no one would notice that I *hadn't* just come from the sluice. Casually I picked up the chart, noted 6 oz. and looked up to meet Sister's penetrating gaze.

'Glad to see you're keeping this up to date,' said the charming Mr Prentiss, taking it from my grasp. 'They're very important you know, Nurse.'

He launched into one of his impromptu rehearsals for the nurses' surgical lectures. I listened politely, though itching to get back to my stopped drip and kidney dish of aspiration. Still, he was always so nice and polite to everyone, even addressing himself to junior nurses!

At last I escaped. Now, which should I do? Empty the dish and measure aspiration, and be accused of not noticing the stopped drip, while also reducing the chances of getting it going again? Or fix the drip, only to be told off for being late with the aspiration and leaving it lying around in that unhygienic manner? When Sister's back was turned I did a crafty compromise. I guessed the amount of aspiration, which was fairly easy, stuck the nasty stuff behind the curtain on the window sill and noted it on the chart.

Now I could be earnestly engaged in first aid on the drip when they arrived. I undid the control clip, made sure the tube wasn't kinked, milked it, loosened the bandages around the arm, moved the needle very slightly and gently stroked the vein—all to no avail. No puffiness in the surrounding tissues, so it probably wasn't leaking.

The entourage arrived, the houseman cursed under his breath and took over the fiddling. He made sure there were no kinks in the tube, milked it, checked that the bandages were not too tight, moved the needle slightly, stroked the vein and finally disconnected the giving set from the needle and flushed it through, all to no avail.

He groaned. 'It's the needle or the vein; I suppose I'll have to cut down. Keep trying, Nurse, I'll come back in a minute.' He looked very weary; he'd been up half the night again.

'Better set up a cut-down trolley, Nurse—just in case,' Sister said over her shoulder as they moved on.

'But, Sister, I've never——' She was gone. Sister was usually very good about making sure we could do what she requested.

I had another try at getting the drip going—oh, it was a waste of time—I'd better measure the aspiration, then go and grovel to someone to help me with the trolley.

I collected Mr Spencer's gastric juices from behind the curtain and cursed; the third blood was due *and* Mr Lowrie's next aspiration. What a bloody awful job this was—why should I worry myself to death just because they were too mean to give us enough nurses to cope? I could pack it all in and——

'It's going again, Nurse,' said Mr Spencer proudly.

By Jove, it was too—racing in fact. I'd left the clip undone—quick, slow it down before it flooded. Wow, that was a relief. I whispered the good news to the houseman.

'Clever girl,' he sighed with a wan smile.

Praise indeed! I danced away with the aspiration; I was almost up-to-date with my work now. I gave Mr Slack a bottle for his urine specimen.

'Can't find anyone out here,' said the nicer porter, popping his head round the door. 'Where do you want this emergency?' He indicated the sorry-looking occupant of his trolley.

I led the way to the deposed Mr Rose's bed.

'It's stopped again, Nurse,' said Mr Spencer apologetically.

'Nurse!' interrupted Mr Slack urgently, 'Mr Wartski doesn't look too good—he's gasping!'

'You're late, dear,' said my mother as I joined her in the dining-room. 'Been busy?'

'Average.'

Normally, I wouldn't have sat with the third-years but there was a spare seat and they had invited me to join my mother. They tolerated my presence occasionally as my mother was popular—she mothered all of them—but they had been strangely eager for me to join them today.

'Where are you now?' one asked, being polite.

'She's on Fieldman,' broke in Male Nurse James coyly.

'Oh, condolences.'

'I don't know, I think people exaggerate about Fieldman, don't you? Out Patients is much harder,' pouted Nurse Withers, who was safely off Fieldman and working guess where?

I nodded vaguely, so as to avoid antagonizing anyone.

Why was everyone watching me? There was an oddly tense atmosphere at the table; they all seemed to be sharing a private joke. It was becoming irritating.

'You're a naughty girl,' said my mum. 'You forgot to put the milk bottles out when you left.' (I had slept at home the previous night after my day off.)

'Oh, sorry. Were there any letters?'

'No.'

Male Nurse James looked puzzled. 'What's all this about milk bottles and letters—do you two live together, or something?'

At this all eyes widened and lips tightened in barely suppressed mirth which was suddenly unleashed as my mum said innocently, 'Oh, haven't you met my daughter?'

His face registered utter astonishment, then he blushed furiously. Everyone screamed with laughter and fell about, except Male Nurse James and me. He was furious, jumped up from his seat, exclaiming, 'I don't know what's so funny!' and stalked off.

This was the signal for more hysterics during which they enlightened me in little, gasping sentences. As I had entered the dining-room and looked for Bill's letter on the sideboard, Male Nurse James had confided in my mother that I was the one he had his eye on at the moment. The others had held their breath and listened in growing disbelief, while he had discussed my attributes in great detail. It seemed he was the only one there who did not know we were related—heaven knows why. No wonder the sadists had been eager for me to join them—and I had thought I was becoming popular!

It was my nineteenth birthday and we were erecting beds in Fieldman's corridor. We had already squeezed enough beds down the sides and the centre of the two male wards to make the area of space recommended for each patient a joke. Now there were two in the corridor between the kitchen and sluice: just a temporary arrangement, we were assured. But we didn't really mind as they gave the ward a gay, camping-out atmosphere. Also we knew that no matter how hard we tried we would never get through all the work and this brought a certain acceptance and relief of tension. And we were less bothered by the needs of the average patient. They soon realized that unless they were emergencies, critically ill or dying, they could not claim much of our attention. Every mobile person mucked in uncomplainingly—happily in fact, for they felt needed. They knew that if they did not make the mid-morning milky drink there would be no mid-morning milky drink. We were comrades in arms: the blitz all over again.

Some patients may have gone home exhausted, but certainly not dying of boredom. Even many of the bed-bound seemed to thrive on the dramatic, life-and-death atmosphere. Interest in the outcome of the struggle for survival kept their minds alert, reduced the importance of their own ailments and made them do as much as possible for themselves. The biggest drawback, as always on Fieldman, was the difficulty in getting sufficient sleep, what with the constant activity day and night.

But about this time a new type of patient became more obvious to me: the spoiled. Very ill patients still received excellent constant care—even more than usual, since our trivial tasks were alleviated by the other patients. We, and the ward, were inclined to make pets of them and get deeply involved in their fate. But as soon as they were out of danger and well on their way, they had to join the others in fending for themselves. And some did not like it. In fact, they were our only fractious patients. Their hour of trial had also been their hour centre-stage: they'd been really important for a while. When we were behind the screens tending their successors, we could hear them boring new arrivals with the harrowing details of how they had 'nearly died' and how concerned everyone had been. One particular man, who had been the darling of us all when struggling to hold his own because of his uncomplaining, cheerful stoicism, astonished us by 'turning' when he was getting better.

But one who didn't turn was Mr Wartski. He'd gone down for the third time and come up again nodding and smiling and with a new phrase, 'How are you today?'. He was thriving now and would soon be returning to his ship. We would miss him.

A telegram for me was delivered to the ward: 'Happy Birthday from an ardent admirer.' Who on earth could that be? Then I laughed. I knew who it was—Mr Slack and Co.

That morning, when someone told them it was my birthday, they insisted on leading the ward in a painful rendition of 'Happy Birthday to you' and were disappointed to hear that at the moment there was no current boy-friend to take me out on the town to celebrate. So they had invented an admirer. They must have gone to a lot of trouble to send it—how sweet.

I went in to inform them I'd called their bluff and to thank them. There were screens around their beds but, carried away with the sentiment, I ignored them and pushed through.

'Thank you for the telegram,' I said, grinning.

'What telegram?' said Mr Slack, but seemed disinclined to continue the conversation, which wasn't surprising; even an ardent admirer loses his aplomb when sitting on a bedpan.

About this time I chose to catch tonsillitis; the verb 'to catch' is particularly apt here, as it suggests deliberate intention. Nurses always caught things deliberately, if they were not merely imagining they had caught them. All the compassion we were urged to extend to the sick somehow never applied to us.

One of my colleagues had hobbled with a broken ankle for several days because a cursory examination by a casualty officer had failed to diagnose correctly. Another suffered for some months the classic swelling of neck and bulging eyes of thyrotoxicosis until my mother pointed out the obvious (although, to be fair, instead of the usual over-activity typical in such patients, he was positively lethargic). And at least three had to practically collapse before examination revealed that they had been inconsiderate enough to contract tuberculosis (Nurse Sinclair was one).

But where labour was at such a premium and replacements impossible to find, even we nurses sometimes felt resentment, doubt and even envy when one of our colleagues went sick and left us holding the syringe. And it *is* true that nurses are hypochondriacs—no, that's not fair, it's just that they tend to over-estimate the importance of their symptoms. So many cases of colic, nausea, etc., that they see in hospital turn out to be appendicitis or 'perfs.' and not the more common upsets caused by mild infection or self-abuse, as is the case in the domestic scene. So, that's what they think of first. In fact, they almost begin to believe that the serious diagnosis is more common; it is, in fact, to them.

As a layman you might be forgiven for supposing that my acute follicular tonsillitis was encouraged by my being tired and over-worked when a particular bug decided to come-a-calling. But Matron was a woman of wider experience. When I returned and reported back she lectured me on the duty of a nurse to maintain her health with adequate sleep, food and warm clothing.

'I suppose,' she accused, 'you wear those silly, sleeveless vests!'

I hadn't the nerve to admit that I didn't wear a vest at all, so I confessed to the former, which seemed to satisfy her. Now that I had accepted full responsibility for my illness I was allowed to return to the ward and expiate my guilt.

CHAPTER VIII

Night-Duty Medley

Nights on medical were fairly easy. There was the odd emergency admission such as a heart failure or a stroke, and one could never avoid the evening and early morning rush to 'get done', but compared with the ever-hectic Fieldman or Smithfield, which sometimes reeled under the day's heavy list and a couple of bad accidents, it was a piece of cake.

The senior girl soon went back to days and I, with my vast experience of medical, was left in charge—with Nurse Foxley as my junior. That was lucky; it was murder spending the night with someone one didn't like, or a junior with whom one had to go to endless lengths in order to hide one's ignorance. I couldn't kid Foxley; indeed, she would have been rather disappointed if I'd suddenly become efficient, so we mucked in together.

The male patients were a nice lot this time. Two or three jolly younger ones set the tone and the atmosphere was great. We night staff were pets; night staff always tended to 'belong' to the patients more than day staff did. We got on particularly well and on arrival every evening did a lap of honour to greet our loyal subjects.

They were generous to a fault, and heaped sweets and choco-lates on us—especially Mr Callington, a tall, handsome and very masculine gall bladder, who seemed to want to give me his all. But, despite being somewhat smitten, all else he could think about was 'getting out of this place'. He was the type that went on and on about it, so although sorry to lose him we were quite relieved when he finally got his marching orders. *He* was delighted.

Three of the men were suffering from inoperable cancer of the lung. Fortunately they had no idea, were quite cheerful and, apart from being somewhat 'chesty', were quite comfortable. Mr Arlington and Mr Foster, who slept opposite each other, were special long-term favourites, with a cheerful camaraderie in their shared symptoms.

We had no intravenous drips to watch during the night, but we did have two gastric ulcers with milk drips *in situ*. Though the flow of milk down the nasal tube to the stomach had to be kept going continuously, our observation on them was not as critical as the other kind. Running dry meant a slight slacking off in the neutralizing of stomach acid, not a likelihood of allowing air into a vein.

Night Sister would come quietly up the stairs to see if she could catch us with our caps off and our aprons undone. On the long, mostly undisturbed nights on medical we would sit over the plate warmer in the kitchen and read, write letters and rack our brains over the night report. As the night wore on the discomfort of the starchy waistband and the irritation of trying to avoid a mashed cap when sitting in a high-backed armchair would become too tiresome and we would yield to temptation. This was a crime because it meant that we weren't 'ready for an emergency', Sister said: all it really meant though was that we were not ready for Sister. We were quite capable of fastening and donning at the run and anyway I doubt whether the shock of seeing a capless nurse would have seriously endangered any patient's life.

But not hearing her sneak up the stairs was also a crime—it meant we were asleep. If we didn't hear *her*, we wouldn't hear all the patients moaning and dying, all too far gone to press their bells. Both counts were federal offences, so our hearing became acute and we took turns in loosening aprons and removing caps so that one of us was always ready to dash out and stall Sister.

But we were surprised one night when our antennae picked up noises on the stairs when even Sister shouldn't be sneaking about. She had just been and, according to the rules of the game, should be just settling down for her cuppa and should only be disturbed by surgical emergencies, heart attacks or aborting women on Pilkington Ward. Doctor had visited very early on and we were not expecting any admissions.

Puzzled, I peered out to see a blue-suited figure swaying slightly at the top of the stairs. As I approached, the figure became vaguely familiar—ridiculous—it couldn't be! But yes it was—Mr Callington who had been discharged a week ago.

'What on earth are you doing here?' I exclaimed.

He grinned with foolish delight on seeing me, emitted waves of beery breath and loudly announced to an imaginary audience, 'I've come back!' If watery eyes can be said to mist over, his did. 'I miss you all and I've come back to stay!'

Having issued his proclamation, he pointed himself in the general direction of the men's ward and began wobbling determinedly towards it. I hissed for Foxley who, having presumed the male voice to be that of the porter come to check the oxygen cylinders, had stayed in her cosy armchair. Our minds froze at the awfulness of the situation. I liked him and didn't want to see him in trouble; on the other hand, I knew if we tried to handle it on our own and got caught, everyone would believe the worst. What a seedy drama they could make of this! Still, even if we reported it, we knew from experience that the fault would turn out to be ours; so what the hell, we might as well have a go. Our horror-struck expressions and the urgency in our voices managed to convey something of the seriousness of the situation to Mr Callington's befuddled brain, and to persuade him that he could not sleep here. He was rather hurt by the cold reception; the bosom of the family was not welcoming the prodigal son.

'All right, then,' he finally agreed in a stage whisper. 'Just let me go and see old Bob and then I'll go.'

We shushed him madly and dragged him into the kitchen, thus getting ourselves in deeper if we were caught. In the *kitchen*! (You can make anywhere sound sinful if you really try.) Margaret sneaked down the stairs to see if the way was clear and to warn the staff in the ward below to keep out of sight. I stayed in the kitchen with Mr Callington who was now becoming maudlin and, inflamed by the intimacy of the situation, was whispering sweet nothings to me. To keep him occupied and stop him wandering off to see old Bob, I engaged him in conversation.

'How did you get as far as this without being seen?' I asked. I was really curious anyway.

He humoured me and chanted patiently, 'Through the front door, along the corridor and up the stairs,' in a tone which suggested, how else?

Foxley's hoarse whisper, 'All clear', came from the top of the stairs so I escorted him there while she crept down again, peered around furtively, and beckoned us on. At the bottom of the stairs we aimed him in the right direction, crossed our fingers that his luck would hold and left him. If he was caught now we would have to disclaim all knowledge. We panted upstairs again to pray and watch his shaky progress off the grounds. He made it and I never saw him again.

As soon as the curtains were drawn back and the lights clicked on to augment the struggling dawn, mad activity commenced. The dark and peaceful silence was shattered by clattering basins in the sink, with Foxley shouting, 'Wakey, wakey!' to herald the start of the wash round.

We were going to be busy this morning—several patients to

prepare for lab. tests and X-ray examinations. I was doing the steadier temperatures round which was much more suitable for the delicate way I felt. But it was still a difficult enough job, trying to wake them sufficiently to make them open their mouths to accept the thermometer without closing them again with a crunch. One also had to watch for the physically-obedient-but-still-asleep types who would open sesame at a touch but leave their jaw dropped, like a ball receptacle at a fairground stall, then lean forward, yawning, and deposit the thermometer on the floor.

At last Mr Casement stirred, yawned, but kept his eyes tightly shut. I immediately pushed a thermometer into the gaping chasm that was his mouth, closed it manually and shouted dire threats into his closed face of the consequences, should he let it fall.

Mr Foster was being very naughty. People who slept sitting up, as he did 'for his chest', always looked as though they were only pretending to sleep anyway. I gave him another irritable shake and was tempted to risk putting the thermometer into his open but inert mouth when something about the quality of his stillness finally penetrated my sluggish grey matter. He wasn't breathing. In fact he was sitting there as large as life, but very dead.

I was stunned, for although his condition had been deteriorating he certainly hadn't seemed anywhere near death. I felt very sad as I'd liked him. Sudden death, with its lack of preparation and goodbyes, is odd, unfinished. But I was glad for his sake—no lingering or pain. Though I must admit that these noble thoughts came upon me later. Right at that moment a more urgent, selfish thought was uppermost. It was obvious that he hadn't just died when we put the lights on. He'd been dead for some time so we'd committed one of the three cardinal sins: letting a patient die (without finding out about it sooner, that is). The others are: 'letting a patient fall out of bed' and 'letting a patient get bedsores'. And last night I'd been caught without a cap and apron, thus confirming Sister's suspicion that I slept all night.

Although we knew we were not guilty, that didn't stop us acting as if we were. Even in the daylight he'd appeared to be asleep so, short of flashing a light in his eyes and shaking him, I didn't see how we could have discovered his condition anyway. But nevertheless we knew that 'That will not do, Nurse'.

What a nuisance he was so bent up. I hoped we'd be able to straighten him out. We daren't do it till Sister and Doctor had been, but popped in a few hot-water bottles in an attempt to warm him up a bit. We rehearsed our stories and excuses, though we doubted whether we'd be allowed a hearing, and awaited Sister with growing guilt complexes. She had sounded suspicious on the phone.

Twenty minutes later she still hadn't come, and in our imaginations Mr Foster grew stiffer and stiffer. Then she rang to say she was held up by a life and death struggle on Pilkington Ward and Staff would be along in a minute.

Five minutes later Staff flew in and flew out again saying, Yes, he was dead. We were duly impressed by this information which Dr Harmsworth, in a gay, tartan dressing gown, sleepily reaffirmed a few minutes later. Neither seemed even slightly interested in why we hadn't discovered him earlier. It was quite an anti-climax and, to cap it all, Mr Foster straightened out like a dream. He did put us right behind with our work though.

The rest of the patients got rather tired of being peered at for the next few nights, and were relieved when we got bored with it and left them to die in peace.

After Mr Foster's death, Mr Arlington lost his gaiety and began to get depressed. 'He had the same as me,' he insisted. In vain we lied in our teeth, claiming Mr Foster had suffered from a dreaded rare disease, and reducing Mr Arlington's to bronchitis.

It didn't help when Mr Burrows, the other cancer of the lung, died during the night in a most distressing manner. Fluid collected continuously in his pleura faster than we could drain it off, making him feel as if he was drowning, which he was really. Eventually his heart gave up the struggle, but it was ghastly while it lasted.

Mr Burrows was at the other end of the ward, almost out of sight of Mr Arlington, so we hoped he would not realize. But his depression grew and he was persistently asking to be put into a single room for some peace and quiet. We kept stalling, as no one thought it a very good idea, but eventually his request was granted. As we expected, he grew more melancholy and often asked, 'I am dying, aren't I, Nurse?' or, 'Have I got cancer?'

To lie consistently about these things is difficult. He pressured me in particular as, after the gay camaraderie of the night staff with the men's ward, he felt I was a friend and would not only care but also tell him the truth. Sometimes he decided to believe me and cheered up for a while, but I avoided having long chats with him.

Finally, he became adamant and insisted he had a right to know and would, in fact, feel better if he knew for certain one way or another. I thought he might be right. With relatives' permission, an appointment was fixed for an interview with the doctor.

When I arrived for duty on the day of the interview, Sister told me that Mr Arlington had not spoken since he had been told, but just lay like a zombie. I dreaded going in to see him. I just couldn't go in on my usual quick, preliminary round and ask, 'How are you today?' But soon I had to answer his bell. He was lying hunched up, facing away from the door. He turned his head as I entered.

'I *am* dying, Nurse Driscoll,' he said quietly.

It was one of the worst moments of my young life. What could I say? I struggled for words. My stock phrases 'Don't be silly' and 'Of course you're not' stood me in little stead now. He took pity on me.

'It's no use telling me this time that I'm not, Nurse. They told me today.'

'I'm sorry,' I stammered.

He smiled wanly and turned his face away again.

He sank into a deep melancholy from which he never recovered whilst I was on the ward. It would have been better if he had not known.

'Fine, thank you,' said Mrs Evelyn, that evening's threatened abortion, in answer to my dutiful enquiries.

'Well, the moment you feel anything, ring me,' I ordered.

The senior nurse was having her nights off and I was in sole charge of Pilkington, the gynaecological ward, a newly frightening responsibility, partly due to the likes of Mrs Evelyn.

But threatened abortion was not quite as dramatic as it sounds. For some reason, the word abortion had come to convey induced miscarriage (at that time, criminally), when in fact it just meant miscarriage.

We had several variations on the theme. 'Threatened' merely meant what it said. We would try to save the baby by keeping the mother rested, etc., but any minute she might abort. Other types were: 'incomplete', when the patient had aborted but 'products of conception' remained in the uterus, often causing continuous haemorrhage; 'missed', when the embryo had died but remained *in situ* until expelled or surgically removed; 'inevitable' was—inevitable. It hadn't yet but it would, because the cervix was dilated or part of the foetal membrane had been passed; 'complete' and 'septic' are self-explanatory.

These cases, often in an acute condition, would appear at any time of the day or night, bringing hectic activity in their wake. Any of them *could* be the result of criminal interference but it was so often difficult to tell and no one seemed to waste much time trying to find out. In later years, when serving as a police officer, my report, in which I used the medical 'threatened abortion' instead of a lay term such as possible miscarriage, sent a C.I.D. officer rushing round to the hospital to uncover dastardly plots.

I was busy that night. It had been an op. day and I had a couple of majors to look after. I was well behind, but struggling through, when Mrs Evelyn rang.

'Sorry to bother you, Nurse, but I think something's happened. I feel a bit damp.'

'Let's have a look, dear.'

I pulled back the sheets. 'Something' had indeed happened. There, in the bed, lay the foetus and a lot of blood.

It was a startling experience to see the minute embryo baby, tiny fists clenched and eyes tightly shut, perfect in every detail, lying there in its transparent sac. Mrs Evelyn seemed quite unaware of what had happened.

'Did you have a pain?' I asked.

'Oh no, only a bit uncomfortable.'

'Well, just keep still, dear. Don't move about, I won't be a minute.'

She looked fine and quite unworried. I wasn't though. I rang Sister, who came quickly, examined her and peered at the mess between the sheets.

'I'm afraid you've lost it, dear,' she told Mrs Evelyn. Then to me, 'It seems to be all there. You can clear it up, Nurse, but save it all for the doctor to see.'

'Yes, Sister.' Lucky old him, I thought.

When clearing it up, I had cause to be grateful for the full-length rubber sheets that were always placed under the ordinary sheets in this ward. Previously, I had thought them a bit much and had ignored it when I had seen patients sneaking them off at night.

Mrs Evelyn seemed quite resigned to her loss and accepted it without a frown—if she was *Mrs* Evelyn that is. Often we never knew whether the girl was married or whether the baby was wanted, which made it a little bit awkward when they lost them. The ones who wanted them would try to be stoical whilst those who didn't would try not to look too joyous. But those admitted for threatened abortion usually wanted to save their pregnancy, or they wouldn't be there.

The rest of the work on this ward involved a variety of gynae. conditions. The operations performed were new to me and had some very odd and unpronounceable names.

There were what were loosely termed, 'the plastics', such as anterior colporrhaphy, posterior colpoperineorrhaphy and the more homely Fothergill's and Gillian's, which were all concerned with repairing or excising bits that were giving way and shoring them up again.

The women, not unnaturally, found these names difficult to digest and were much happier with, 'I've had a plastic, Nurse.' The trouble was that some of them really thought they had bits of plastic inside them and would say, 'I've got a plastic inside, Nurse, will I still get a thrill?'

The remainder were mainly hysterectomies, salpingectomies (removal of fallopian tube), oophorectomies (removal of ovary) salpingo-oophorectomies (now you can guess that one) and numerous D. and C.'s (dilatation and curettage of the uterus for diagnosis, treatment, or the removal of those retained products of conception after an abortion).

'You'll get one of three answers, if you ask them what they've had done,' laughed a relieving houseman one night. '"A plastic", "I've been scraped" or "I've had everything taken away".'

He was right, too. But what was more surprising was that so few of the women knew what they had had in the first place, and had even less idea of what they had left. What's more, they didn't seem that interested. But I think our education and the attitudes of the medical profession have a lot to do with this. Have you noticed how Australian dentists are less concerned with conserving their omnipotence and dignity, and manage to explain what they are doing, without being mystical or patronizing?

Although we were dealing mainly with such intimate anatomy, it was treated just like any other medicine, and I never saw any sniggering (there were no students) or indeed any embarrassment; well, except once.

We were blessed with an exceedingly handsome, shy and hesitant houseman. He certainly proved a distraction for the patients and staff, who ogled him and showed great interest in his private life. His fiancée, another doctor, was tall, plain to a degree and looked very strong in character. He ('they' said) was mad about her, but she was not so fussy and had recently broken off their engagement. But after his entreaties she had relented and it was on again.

One evening he apologized to us in his sweet way—he had not been able to get round earlier to examine that day's admissions, so did we mind. . . . We did, as it would tie up one of us when we should have been 'getting on', but he was so nice. . . .

The first on the list was Mrs Middleton, a bubbly, curly haired brunette. She watched Dr Manston's handsome face closely as he asked her questions and pressed gently on her abdomen, trying to detect any signs of rigidity or lumps. Then he slipped on his rubber glove to do the usual vaginal examination. The atmosphere was clinical and he was as serious and dedicated as always, though a sight too slow for my liking. We'd never get the lights out at this rate.

With a frown of concentration on his face, he commenced his digital examination. Suddenly, Mrs Middleton let out a gasp of ecstasy: 'Oh Doctor!' she sighed, and grasped his arm. The look of utter astonishment on his face was followed rapidly by wild blushing embarrassment. He finally managed a 'Now, now Mrs Middleton' in what was meant to be a steadying tone. He finished his examination in record time and, with a parting 'I'll do the rest in the morning, Nurse, it's getting late', fled the ward.

Good, we could get on now.

Pilkington was very hard work, especially on op. mornings, with preparatory catheterizations, douches and bowel washouts. And I needed my sleep.

I was not getting enough in the nurses' home; the cleaners were a noisy lot. Also I was fed up with the eternal rules and regulations, the inquisitive and tell-tale cleaners and the impertinent inspection rounds by Home Sister, who even looked in our wardrobes and chests of drawers to see if they were tidy—and this in our absence! But going home took such a long time. So when Heather, who was slightly junior to me, suggested we take digs nearby I accepted with alacrity.

The digs—one ground-floor room—seemed pleasant enough at first. But soon the snags became apparent, especially for day-time sleeping. The street, which had seemed quiet when we first saw it in the evening, came alive with traffic during the day. It had quite a gradient and lorries found it necessary to change down just outside our room.

The food, quite good at first, soon deteriorated and became sparse and stodgy. The husband began to take an undue interest in us fresh young things, which didn't please his wife too much. One day when I had finally got to sleep I awoke with a start to find her in my room—just standing and looking at me!

Upstairs lived the ex-patient who had arranged the digs. She was one of those people who are totally in love with their illness and was overjoyed to have two captive nurses on the premises. We were waylaid at every opportunity and treated to graphic descriptions of her symptoms.

All in all, living out was a total failure, but we couldn't back out yet. We had had to fight too hard for the privilege and couldn't bear their 'told you so's' to be too triumphant. Anyway, we'd look for somewhere else first.

My heart sank when I read, 'Nurse Driscoll to Heathcote'. I thought I'd managed to avoid the dreaded nights on the geriatric and chronic ward. It was a hardship posting and no one stayed on it for long. Everyone told me how awful it was, but when one has been well prepared for something it is often not as bad as one expects. Heathcote was not as bad as they said: it was worse.

On my first night I was in charge again, even though I didn't know the ward or any of the patients. The Day Staff Nurse took me around to give me some idea. She stopped at the first patient.

'This is our Mrs Parker. How are you, Mrs Parker?' she enquired.

No answer.

'Mrs Parker?'

No answer.

'Oh dear, I think she's dead.'

Surprise, surprise, I thought suspiciously, and oh my God, as well as finding my way round the patients and getting through the ridiculous amount of work before lights out, we now had a body. It was an omen.

The ward was old and decrepit, with echoing, wooden floors and high windows providing no view. There were too many patients for us to look after and they were all old and/or chronically sick. They needed an inordinate amount of care. There were incontinents, colostomies, night wanderers and those in the last stages of debilitating diseases or senile decay. What's more they were so bloody awful to nurse.

Stripped of the veneer of civilization by old age, disease, boredom, their awful surroundings and a feeling of being forgotten and neglected naturally brought out the worst in them. They were carping and self-obsessed. Some were deliberately vicious and would tell tales of our real or supposed omissions to the Day Sister, who listened.

I would come off the ward in the mornings so exhausted that I could hardly stand and so depressed that I wanted to cry. My abortive attempt at living out did not help. I was always late getting off so couldn't get to bed before the lorries started, but I was usually too strung up to go to sleep anyway so I began to take some Soneryl and Sonalgin tablets left over from the patients. Sometimes they beat the lorries and sometimes they didn't and made me feel worse. I was glad when my mother put her foot down and insisted I went home. I was gladder still when my stint on geriatric finished, and I vowed never to go near one of the beastly places again as long as I lived.

CHAPTER IX

Mostly Wendover

Back on days, I was also back on theatre. But gynae. theatre this time, situated in a poky room leading off the end of Pilkington. To reach it the surgeon and staff had to pass back and forth through the ward, which must have been a bit unnerving for the patients, though it did make theatre staff and their fancy dress a familiar sight and thus less fearsome when their turn came. And it was very convenient for us to be able to pop them straight back into bed so quickly.

The list started with the D. and C.'s which, like the tonsils at the Ear, Nose and Throat Hospital, were ten a penny. After a while I became very adept at accepting the dirty D. and C. trolley into the tiny sluice and sterilizing room, giving a sterile one in return, then cleaning and scrubbing the instruments, putting them back into the sterilizers, setting up the next trolley, then exchanging it for a dirty one which I then cleared, and so on. In fact I became too good at organizing this potential chaos, so I kept being given the job. I began to feel like a dreary, wispy little kitchen maid, locked away in my dark steamy little room, whilst my more presentable colleagues were allowed to mix with the clientele!

But it was an intimate theatre with a pleasant atmosphere. The only thing to which I never became accustomed was the position of the patients for the D. and C. and one or two other ops. Lichotomy it was called. They lay on their backs, legs akimbo, supported below the knees by slings; it looked so indecorous, crude in fact. Of course, they were under anaesthetic so it didn't bother them!

Wendover

'I've had a letter from my friend; she's gone into the Wyndham Hospital,' said Mrs Arbour. Then, lowering her voice, 'Poor thing must have *cancer*—they only take cancer there, don't they, Nurse?' She uttered the dread word with reluctant horror.

'Sorry about your friend, Mrs Arbour, but they can recover, you know. I'm afraid I don't know the hospital, though.' I didn't either, but I did know that Mrs Arbour was suffering from cancer of the uterus. I wondered why it had never occurred to her—or perhaps it had.

After another spell on general surgical, I had been transferred to Wendover, another gynae. ward. Wendover did not touch the minor gynae. like D. and C.'s, nor any 'plastics', but dealt mainly with major gynae. surgery or treatments for fibroids, cysts and cancer. The surgeon, who was in sole charge, was considered an expert in his field and people came from all over the country for his treatment, especially when the op. was likely to be difficult or extensive. This meant that visiting was different from the rest of the hospital—fewer times per week but longer, especially on Sundays.

A bright, airy ward on the second floor, Wendover was divided into two. One section was used mainly for those staying one or two nights for a preliminary examination or a follow-up check, and for those undergoing radium treatment. The other housed the major ops.

The frequent use of radium put the staff at some risk, so from time to time we were supplied with two radium indicators (the size and shape of lighter-fuel sacs) which we wore around our necks in little cloth bags for about a fortnight at a stretch. Their purpose was to measure our radiation intake during that period.

The first time I wore mine they swung forward as I was closing the bedpan washer and were crushed between the metal sides! Very occasionally we had blood tests.

The risk to other patients was negated by leaving a lot of space around the beds of those under treatment, and forbidding the other patients to go near them. It is continuous close contact which is risky. One patient had such a massive dose that she was put in a side ward, and we were warned not to spend longer than absolutely necessary either in the room or even in the vicinity. We didn't!

Every morning we checked the rubbish bins with a Geiger counter before we allowed their removal, just in case the minute radium needles had worked loose and got into pads or dressings. Not only was it dangerous but also extremely expensive. The small metal box would break into intermittent little stutters when confronted with bedpans or dressings from radium patients, but to show the new girls how it reacted when faced with the real thing, we would take it close to the beds of those who had radium *in situ*, when it would break into wild, staccato stuttering and the needle would swing madly about.

Lots of treatment, such as 'doing the backs' with cream instead of spirit, was different on Wendover because the resident genius had his own very definite ideas about almost everything. He also had a sense of humour, of sorts, which he displayed when the ward staff toilet became blocked (yet again) by a sanitary towel; he threatened to perform wholesale hysterectomies should it re-occur!

Much speculation and comment greeted my arrival on Wendover. My mother had had a spell there and was adored by the patients. I became a little weary of 'If you're half as good as your mother you'll be all right!' 'But,' they assured me, 'she wasn't soft with us—used to tell us off if we got too sorry for ourselves!'

Which was wise of her. Wendover could be a harrowing ward. Though many of the operations for cancer were successful (but always subject to check-ups for several years), there was always a nucleus of failures and some became pitiful wrecks of skin, bone and foul smell before they died. Some developed secondaries of the chest or brain and became deranged. I remember one particular woman in her mid-thirties who insisted on disrobing her still young and attractive body and running into the corridor or kitchen. Eventually she had to be removed to a mental hospital as we could no longer control her. Her disturbed mind did, however, make her happy and gay to a degree, which is more than can be said for many of us, and we hoped that it would help her when she was dying.

The ward taught us a great deal about the strength of the human spirit. Some who might have pulled through just gave up and died. Others who we felt sure could not survive defied us and thrived, whilst those who could not possibly live another hour lived on for days and days.

The genius's prize patient was a remarkable woman. In her mid-thirties, she had undergone just about the most extensive excision possible: uterus, vagina, ovaries, rectum, bladder, urethras and much intestine. Her lower abdomen was completely closed and both her urine and faeces came from the piece of bowel brought out onto her abdomen—a wet colostomy. It was an operation that some nurses admitted they would sooner die than undergo. I met her when she returned to be investigated, as it seemed that her kidneys were being infected through the ureters being implanted in the colon and something was going to have to be done about it. She was gay, cheerful, very smart and supported by a handsome, loving husband. The genius had photographs of her looking svelte and spry, despite the colostomy bag she was required to wear. It was said he showed them to Americans and Scandinavians when he visited and lectured in their countries. She was philosophical about this new setback—after all, she'd been granted one extension of life and that was something, wasn't it? A remarkable woman.

The women in the ward showed their usual vagueness about their ailments, though in some cases this may have been a defence mechanism. They were also very inclined to boredom. Being mostly wives and mothers, with the sapping of individuality and mental development that these conditions encourage, especially in northern working-class areas, they had no resources apart from a bit of knitting. Few read books and even fewer had any conversational topic apart from our Jimmy's girl and how Bert was managing. We heard none of the male patients' queries, such as 'Why are you changing that drip from blood to saline?' or 'What's that supposed to do?' when giving an injection. Admittedly this was a relief to us—the relentless, know-all patient can be a pain—but the total lack of intelligent interest did reflect sadly on the brain-atrophied second sex.

I bent the hot-water bottle over to expel the steam, screwed in the stopper and popped the bottle into my capacious uniform pocket. It was a very cold day and I was not going to freeze in my silly cotton dress. The voluminous theatre gown I was to don for doing the dressings would hide the bulge.

I knew I had been given the dressings to do (instead of preps or treatments) only because one of Sister's favourites was off-duty and another helping in the radium theatre: otherwise I never had the chance. Like everything else on Wendover, dressings were inclined to be different. The first was Mrs Hanning, a vulvectomy. A large, triangular-shaped piece of flesh had been excised from her lower abdomen, leaving the area raw. But it was remarkable how quickly it had begun to fill up with healthy, granulating tissue, though it still looked pretty awful. Nurse Challoner sat her on a bedpan and I poured a warm solution of Eusol over the area. It bubbled on contact. With a swab on forceps I carefully wiped away the patches of pus, finished off with a saline rinse, then cleaned and dried the area completely.

'You're very thorough,' commented Nurse Challoner as we moved on. 'The others don't take half that trouble—just pour the stuff over. I'm glad I've got the chance to do it with you, so that I learn the proper way.'

I laughed but I was secretly pleased at this vindication.

Nurse Challoner and I were friends. I had been told before I met her that she was 'very popular with the patients'. That had made me wary. It often meant that the other staff flogged away doing more than their fair share of the dirty work while the saint was busy chatting and 'being popular'.

But Nurse Challoner worked quite well and though at first her flattery and flashing charm made me back away mentally, when she launched her campaign to make a friend of me I was putty in her hands, like everyone else. No one had ever before taken the trouble to charm me.

I was rather pleased that the next patient was due for removal of some stitches. I was very good at removing stitches painlessly, though I expected Mrs Woodward would find something to complain about; she generally did.

Although Mrs Woodward, a strapping Scot, had undergone a much more serious and extensive operation than had at first been expected, I think it fair to say that the results were even more traumatic for the staff. They certainly left a lasting impression on me. At first she had been the life and soul of the ward: gay, saucy, full of jokes, taking everything in her stride and keeping up the other patients' spirits. If only we had more like her we said, she was a *one*, was Mrs Woodward! Until the operation. From then on it was like *The Picture of Dorian Gray*, but personality-wise. From being our best-ever patient she became one of our worst-ever. Not another spark of humour came from her;

she whined, carped, complained, wallowed in self-pity and refused to do anything to help herself. We couldn't believe it. True, it had been a bad op. but lesser souls went through it far more stoically. So we didn't spend longer than necessary with Mrs Woodward.

'You're very good at taking out stitches,' said Nurse Challoner.

Poor Mrs Ince next. Now she really tried to keep her pecker up. A jolly, chubby Yorkshirewoman, she had been very ill after her operation but had begun to recover. The only thing holding her back now was her abdomen. It had become so huge. Distension was not uncommon after gynae. ops. but usually disappeared gradually after the first three or four days, when the bowel started working properly. Mrs Ince's bowel started working all right but the distension remained and it was beginning to get her down.

'You going to dress my balloon?' she grinned, adding with a sigh: 'Wouldn't like to prick it while you're at it, would you?'

It was just a straightforward replacement of a dry dressing. As I cleaned around the stitches, I noticed a little soft patch in the lower half of the incision. Confident and bold after Challoner's praise, I announced, 'There's a soft patch here; I'd better ease it open with the sinus forceps—there's probably a little pus or haematoma underneath.'

Mrs Ince looked worried. She knew I didn't usually do the dressings and didn't need anything else to contend with.

'They don't usually bother with anything like that,' she assured me timidly. 'They just replace the dressing.'

I hesitated. Perhaps I shouldn't muck about if they didn't—what if the whole abdomen should open up under the strain? Oh, what the hell, we were supposed to open these things up and let them drain! The forceps slipped easily into the soft tissues. As they did so, a dark, brownish fluid gushed out and ran all over her abdomen at an alarming rate. I tried to catch it with wads of gauze but they rapidly became saturated.

'*Get Sister!*' I instructed Challoner, quietly but firmly. Mrs Ince looked terrified.

'Don't worry, dear,' I reassured her. 'Looks like this could be the end of your troubles.'

For it was beginning to dawn on me that this might be the reason for her distension: a huge haematoma (pocket of old blood) caused by internal post-op. bleeding. Though it seemed incredible that there could be that much, and also that it had seeped through the muscles and subcutaneous fat to the skin. I was a bit worried too; if it was that big a haematoma, its too rapid release might produce serious shock.

But when Sister arrived it was slowing down to a steady flow. She was surprised but delighted, and even overcame her dislike of me enough to offer a, 'Very good, Nurse Driscoll!'

Three days later Mrs Ince was still seeping and deflating and I had become her heroine. Nurse, Sister, doctors and even the Genius himself had all shaken their heads over her rotundity, but I had just taken one close look and immediately unplugged her. Mrs Ince made sure that all who now came to gaze upon this phenomenon were made fully aware of the fact.

I went off Challoner a bit when I discovered that her charm worked even better on a man, and on my current boy-friend in particular. I'd not been at all enamoured of the boy, but had stuck to him for a while because working hours made it difficult to acquire a replacement. Also he was a genuine university student. This latter fact impressed me greatly, though I couldn't understand why I found him so dull and colourless. Nevertheless I was reluctant to let go of this passport to the intellectual heights and our romance meandered on in desultory fashion. But to see him buckle so readily under the charmer's spell was humiliating.

Now, however, Challoner had her own boy-friend problems and I couldn't help feeling a trifle bitchily pleased. Despite the dozens of men falling over themselves to take her out, she had fallen heavily for Roger, the handsome male nurse, who, it seemed, could take her or leave her. When he did condescend to take her out, she confessed that he was quite content with a very perfunctory goodnight kiss, while she was left panting for a little more. Naturally his lack of susceptibility made her keener than ever.

'Come along, girls,' said Wendover's ample Sister as she sailed along the corridor, 'Mrs Gillie's radium is due out. Come and watch, good experience for you.'

We grinned. That chubby body, Mrs Gillie, was saucy and full of sexy innuendo. She'd only just said to me, 'Doctor's been peeking down our nighties again. Bet he enjoys his job—tickling all those fancies! I showed him mine!'

Four of us trooped in Sister's wake. I'd seen several extractions but it was always useful to see more. Though I was now senior, I usually managed to avoid the insertions which were carried out in the tiny radium theatre. Sister and her close cronies were normally in attendance, which was fine with me. Despite my experience in theatre, swift, adept physical reactions were still foreign to me, and the genius's histrionic carryings-on made my physical impotence complete.

'Coming out at last,' said Sister breezily. 'Ordeal's nearly over.' And pulled back the sheets.

'Thank goodness. You get so sore and uncomfortable lying still for thirty-six hours,' commented Mrs Gillie. But as four of us trooped round the screens, her jolly expression changed to a scowl.

'What do they all want?' she asked belligerently.

'Just to see the radium come out—good experience,' said Sister matter-of-factly as she swabbed down Mrs Gillie.

We waited for the joke which we were sure was coming next.

'Well, I think it's disgusting!' she exploded vehemently. 'All standing there gaping at me. Doesn't one have a right to *any* privacy?' and she glared at us with hate in her eyes.

We were amazed and still waiting for the punch line but it never came—she really meant it. Suddenly, instead of watching a normal extraction, we felt we were being 'not quite nice'. It seemed so ridiculous. We spent much of our working life on Wendover dealing with intimate anatomy. We shaved, prepped for ops., checked radium was *in situ*, douched, dressed wounds, catheterized. It meant absolutely nothing to us. The other women, though sometimes initially shy, realized this and adopted the same attitude. But suddenly Mrs Gillie had made us feel dirty, like some weird peeping-toms. Mrs Gillie of all people —the most sexually outspoken patient we'd ever had!

I give up, I thought—I will *never* understand people.

Thank goodness we still had Mrs Findlay. The radium ward had been going through a bad time lately. First Mrs Felix's mysterious death in the bathroom, and then that cruelly stupid woman telling them they'd all got cancer.

Mrs Felix, who had a probably excisable growth, had gone to the bathroom late one evening. It was during the night staff's busy time, so quite a while elapsed before she was missed. She was found face downwards in a bath which contained a few inches of water. The plug chain was twisted around her neck. It looked like suicide, although she had not seemed depressed or upset previously. It was just possible that she had slipped.

The ward had been brooding more than enough on this when one of the charming patients, in for one-night follow-up tests, having listened to what she felt was their ill-informed chatter, thought fit to tell them not to be silly—they *all* had cancer! They were in a terrible state about it and we had a lot more convincing lies to tell before some sort of equilibrium returned.

But soon after, Mrs Findlay arrived and everything took on a rosier hue. She was one of those people who seem to have their own illumination system. In her early thirties, she was warm, cheerful and full of fun, but with none of the desperate bonhomie of the determined 'life and soul' of the ward. The others gravitated to where she sat and even now, when she lay flat, still and supposedly isolated for her forty-eight-hour radium ordeal, we had to keep shooing them away: such was her magnetism. The wearying treatment did not sap her spirit. She and I had a cosy friendship and I was particularly pleased that she had a good prognosis: her growth had been caught early and appeared easily removable.

Removing radium was not particularly difficult, but had to be done with care and dispatch to avoid harming any tissues and to avoid exposing oneself or the patient to the rays for a second longer than necessary. Also one had to be absolutely sure it was totally removed; if there were several needles and an obscuring pack there was the possibility of leaving some behind. Understandably it was a responsible job, so I was somewhat apprehensive.

Everything went perfectly. Mrs Findlay was delighted to be rid of it and I was very relieved to have retrieved it all. When I confessed that it had been my first extraction she was doubly pleased to have been my guinea pig.

'We must celebrate,' she laughed. 'You did it so beautifully— do take this box of chocolates,' she said, indicating a very swish confection, recently delivered by a doting family.

'Oh no, I couldn't, that's too much!'

'I insist,' she said. 'You'll hurt my feelings if you don't and you know you're not supposed to upset the patients!'

'You win,' I chuckled. 'I'll collect them as I go off duty.'

The following afternoon was warm and sultry. We weren't

very busy and most of the women were having a cosy gossip around Mrs Findlay's bed. I stopped and chatted for a while. As I stirred myself to go, she said, 'Your chockies are still here, Nurse, don't forget them tonight.'

I promised I wouldn't.

Five minutes later a buzzer went in Ward Two. At the same time one of the women popped her head around the sluice door.

'It's Mrs Findlay, Nurse. She's fainted!'

'We've put her back on her bed,' she added as I followed her into the ward.

'But she shouldn't be out of bed yet; she knows that, the naughty girl,' I said, preparing to tell her off.

'She was just slipping out to the toilet. Doesn't like using a bedpan.'

'Well, she's not as strong as she thinks!' I exclaimed as I reached the bed. 'Let's have a look at her then!'

Mrs Findlay was unconscious, her face purple and she was gasping for breath. I couldn't believe my eyes. She looked as though she was choking but though I searched desperately I could find no obstruction in her windpipe.

'Get oxygen and Sister, *quickly*!' I said to the nurse who had followed me into the ward. I turned back to try to help her as she fought for breath, when it struck me like a blow between the eyes—My God—she's dying! Sister was as astonished as I, and said, 'Get Doctor'. But Mrs Findlay was dead.

I was shattered. Mrs Findlay wasn't supposed to die; she was going to be all right, I fumed unreasonably. I had seen death a-plenty but always orderly, expected death, following agradual receding of life, not this rude snatching away of a sparkling personality. It was obscene.

Although I'd never seen anyone die of pulmonary embolism or coronary thrombosis, I guessed it must be one of these. Maybe it was the way I'd taken out her radium—I'd released a clot!

If *I* was shattered, the ward was stunned and broken-hearted. The spirit went right out of them. They just sat and stared at her screened bed in disbelief. I could understand them thinking if she could die any of them could.

It turned out to be coronary thrombosis. The attack may have been precipitated by her getting up after the enforced inactivity, but the tendency was there and it could have happened at any time—no one could tell.

I cleared the usual bits and pieces from her locker: potted plant, make-up bag, books—and a rather swish box of chocolates. Then I locked myself in the toilet and cried.

CHAPTER X

Smithfield Revisited and Night Wandering

Not surprisingly Mrs Withers didn't think it a bit funny to be knocked down by an ambulance. Our attempts to extract some humour from the situation only made it worse.

'Be careful of my leg, Nurse,' she whined, as we gently straightened the sheets over her massive bulk in preparation for visiting time. 'When will it start to get better?' she whimpered for the hundredth time.

But really I didn't blame her. I'd never seen anything quite like her leg. The ambulance concerned had been racing to a call when it lost a wheel, slewed wildly across the road and pinned poor Mrs Withers against a wall. She had suffered such extensive bruising to her thigh that, whilst the fat had probably saved her from a fractured femur, the unhealthy tissue was starting to disintegrate.

The young first-year nurse helping me sang a little hymn to cheer her up.

'Oh, pack it in,' I said a trifle impatiently.

I didn't mind people who'd 'got religion' as long as they didn't keep chucking it around. But Brigitte (she was German) had more than religion. While still patriotically partaking of pumpernickel, she had the strangest passion for all things Scottish, and on her day off would grace the local high street in full Highland regalia—and I mean full! Kilt, sporran, knee-socks, buckled shoes, velvet jacket, lace jabot and tam-o-shanter! I don't remember whether she had a skean-dhu but it seems probable. We pointed out that if she dared to cross the Border in this get-up she would be lynched, and anyway it was hardly *de rigueur* in Bolton or Manchester either. But she thought it attractive and had, at least, the courage of her rather odd convictions.

'Save your breath, darling, I've sold my soul to the devil,' said Jean, the next in line for our roll over, pull through and smooth out routine. She winked at me. She was another of the professional-patient types, transferred from the fever hospital for an operation on her T.B. hip. Jean had hospital living down to a fine art and found it no excuse for slovenliness. Her locker and personal belongings were perfectly organized and her husband was always greeted with full war paint and a crisply laundered blouse: no sloppy nightgowns for Jean.

Roger appeared at the bottom of the bed and glared at Brigitte.

'I'll help old Driscoll,' he said. 'You go and tidy up the lockers and any bedpans that are hanging around. Chop chop. Properly, mind.' Roger was a bit of a fanatic about ward tidiness.

'She's an odd one, that,' laughed Jean as Brigitte trotted off to spread The Word.

'Batty cow,' commented Roger dismissively.

You were either in with Roger or right out. He had no time for people he didn't like. I was now in. Partly, I suspected, because of my oft tiresome habit of standing up for myself, which he admired, and also because of my apparent unshockability. Roger couldn't stand 'pure' types. For my part, I could see his faults but he amused me and I liked him.

'Here, you old bag, who was that young chap I saw you dragging off into the bushes last night?' he asked, exaggerating wildly, but avid for the latest gossip.

Jean pricked up her ears.

'She's a baby snatcher, is she?'

'Oh my dear,' said Roger, raising his eyebrows in mock horror, 'the things I could tell you!'

'Actually, he's quite a lot older than I am—and what's more looks it—you gossipy old busybody. As a matter of fact he's a newspaper reporter,' I added with a hint of pride. One up on a university student in my eyes and much more interesting as a person.

'Gutter press, no doubt,' Roger retorted. 'Hurry up and we can have a drag and a natter before that silly foreign cow gets finished.'

Whilst dragging and nattering amongst the urine testing equipment in the back of the sluice, Roger surprised me by unburdening himself—but lightly of course. I had teased him about his well-documented romance with the charming Challoner.

'She's mad about you, you know. God knows why!' I said rather unfairly.

'I know,' he shrugged ruefully.

'Many blokes would give a lot for your chance.'

'I know,' he admitted again and looked thoughtful. 'Here, Driscoll,' he confided suddenly, 'do you think there's something the matter with me? I don't get a thrill when I kiss a girl good-night—might as well kiss a brick wall!'

'What *you* need,' I advised firmly, 'is a good dose of testo-sterone in your tea!'

'You cheeky old bag!' he laughed.

A bell rang in Ward Two. As I went to answer it, Roger called, 'I'm dashing off to grab a bite of supper. You're in charge. Don't get drunk with power.'

Mr Bernstein was coming out of Ward Two to meet me.

'Come quickly—it's Mr Henry!' he gasped. 'He's having a haemorrhage!'

Oh Lor, and only dear old Brigitte to sustain me. I spotted Mr Henry's pale face craning to see me as I hurried towards him. He was in a near panic.

'Quick, Nurse, you'd better fetch Doctor or something!'

'Turn over and let's have a look,' I said as calmly as possible. Panic can be infectious.

The dressing on his hip wound was saturated with a dark, reddish-brown liquid.

'Relax,' I laughed, 'you're not departing this world yet. It's only a haematoma.'

He looked somewhat relieved but still sceptical. He knew I wasn't usually in charge.

'What's that?' he asked suspiciously.

'Old blood which has collected in a cavity below the surface, and now it's suddenly decided to come out—good thing!'

'Are you sure?'

'Certain.'

'Hadn't you better ask Male Nurse Hinkley?' he ventured.

'No I had *not*!' I snapped. 'I'm quite capable of identifying a haematoma when I see one. Don't be such a big baby. Look, you can see it's old blood—when did you see fresh blood that colour?'

'Sorry,' he grinned and made a ducking movement, 'I was just a bit concerned.'

'Men!' I exclaimed sourly. 'Stay still now while I fetch a new dressing!'

'Yes, *sir*!'

'You'd better hop off to bed now,' I advised Mr Bernstein. 'It's nearly visiting time and these fellows don't deserve your tender care!'

'I'll just get Joe a jug of water before I go,' he said.

'What a nice man he is,' commented a fractured femur, as Mr Bernstein returned to his own ward.

'Humph!' I snorted. 'That's not what you said a week ago!'

'Oh, I was only speaking generally,' he protested. 'Of course there are some nice ones.'

What he had said a week ago was a furtive, 'He's Jewish, you know!'

And when I replied, 'So what?' he had added, 'Can't stand them, not to be trusted'.

Some of the others had nodded their approval of these sentiments.

I was astounded. I'd never met anti-Semitism before; I didn't really know it existed, perhaps because Jews were few and far between in that area, and in hospital so many social barriers certainly seem to be lowered.

I only knew that Mr Bernstein was a very cheery patient. Kind and interested in everything. I had told the men off but they, after shifting uncomfortably, had maintained a smug, 'you'll see' attitude. It transpired that Mr Bernstein did not need me as a champion. Being one of the few mobile patients, he was able and willing to do little jobs for the others. Not only did he make himself useful in his own four-bedded room, but wandered around the other rooms helping out, chatting, always interested and interesting, and above all cheerful. Everyone perked up in his presence and the men soon became eager for his company. They seemed to forget he was a Jew.

'Chicken tonight, Nurse,' said Mr Latham, handing me a greaseproof-paper packet and a large thermos flask.

'Lovely, thanks,' I replied somewhat sheepishly.

Every night Mr Latham handed us the flask and packet of sandwiches containing some delicacy designed to tempt *his* appetite. This was the result of his once complaining to his wife that he had been hungry the previous evening, between the too-early supper and lights out. The following evening the dutiful wife had arrived with a flask of coffee, sandwiches and a home-made pie. He had not been hungry that night, however, and had given them to us. We had enthused over the quality, so every night from then on he had 'felt the need' for extra refreshment. His wife was eager to look after him so everyone was happy, and we felt only slightly guilty as we scoffed them. Mr Latham even insisted on learning our preference, so as to make special requests. It was surprising how welcome the ready-made coffee and food was during or after the evening flog round (about four hours), especially on busy nights when we could pause in turns for a gulp and bite but might not have had the time to make a cup.

We were busy that evening with post-operative cases but at last they were settled. At midnight I had the coffee cup to my lips when the phone rang.

'You've been on Casualty, haven't you, Nurse Driscoll?' enquired the Gipsy Queen, otherwise Night Sister Parrish.

'No, Sister—that's my mother,' I replied for the umpteenth time.

'Oh,' she hesitated, 'still, you can manage, can't you? 'she commanded.

'Yes, Sister.' One didn't argue with the Gipsy Queen.

She was talking to someone beside her. 'Staff Nurse tells me that you *have* done it on nights before,' she said accusingly.

'Yes,' I admitted, omitting to add, 'because Staff Nurse once said, "You've done Casualty before haven't you?" and I said, "No", and she said, "Oh well, you can cope, can't you?"'

I had coped all right, but felt such a fool not knowing the simplest procedures or where anything was.

'Go down straight away—serious accident coming in. Dr Hayes will be there as soon as possible.'

'Yes, Sister.'

Because I had had theatre experience they were used to saying 'Send Nurse Driscoll'. So now it seemed I was going to take on Casualty as well. Still, I often enjoyed it once I got going, and working there made the time fly. At least it wasn't Saturday, the night of the pickled products of punch-ups.

The victim arrived in Casualty at the same time as I did. It had been a bad accident. A young man had been crushed in the cab of his lorry, resulting in multiple injuries and a suspected fractured pelvis. It was possible that his urethra (the tube leading to his bladder) had been severed.

Fortunately, Dr Hayes had followed me in and after a brief examination he decided that the young man should go straight up to the ward. Well, Smithfield were going to be busy after all—they would have their work cut out keeping him alive.

The Gipsy Queen appeared as I was clearing up, and promptly sent me to the theatre to set-up for an appendix and a perf. When the patients and doctors arrived, I dashed around being anaesthetic nurse, swab counter, gown tier and Sister's runner. The atmosphere was much better than daytime theatre—more relaxed and comradely.

One of the more memorable sights of these wee small hours in the theatre was Mr Cartwright on his knees on the floor, black hair even more awry than usual, glasses falling off, sweating, panting and grunting as he wrenched an unconscious man's dislocated hip back into its socket. The leg looked madly weird sticking straight out from the side of his body, and enormous effort and strength were required to bring it back to normal. A greater contrast with fiction's dramatic, delicately skilled operation I can't imagine.

I escorted the patients back to the ward, then returned to plough my way through the chaos until all was pristine once more. It was hard graft on one's own.

Before tidying Casualty I grabbed a brief meal.

When at last I made my way back to Smithfield, a chill dawn light was spreading across the patches of frosted grass between the complex of corridors. Wearily, I pulled my cloak tighter around my thin cotton dress. Oh, for a nice sit down.

'We've been *very* busy!' said the Senior Nurse tartly, as soon as

I entered the ward. 'Never stopped!' Her tone implied that I had been idling or cavorting with the doctors again.

The Junior Nurse dashed by with a pile of basins.

'Wakey, wakey!' she yelled. 'Another bright new dawn awaits you!'

The Gipsy Queen's voice was urgent.

'Go down to Casualty!'

'But, Sister,' I dared to interrupt, 'we're very busy and I'm in charge now. Couldn't Nurse. . .?'

'No! I realize you are busy, but I specially want *you* to do this job for me,' she insisted. 'The ambulance is bringing in a motorcycle accident—I've heard the victims are already dead. We're frantically busy everywhere, and just can't afford the staff to go through all the admission and the laying-out formalities for patients who are dead on arrival. You must speak to Dr Hayes,' she ordered, 'and tell him to examine them in the ambulance. If they are obviously quite dead, then don't allow the ambulance men to dump them on us—they must take them to the local mortuary. On no account allow them to bring the bodies in—if you do they are our responsibility.'

She was no fool and realized only too well the task she was giving me; to request the ambulance men to do anything was enough, but to forbid them to do something was really asking for it. And I didn't like the sound of it all anyway.

I had never heard of this being done, but my experience in Casualty was limited so I could not be sure. I had the feeling it was one of the Gipsy Queen's instant laws. Still, mine was not to reason. . . . I shrugged on my cloak and stalked off to take on the world; drat my reputation.

Dr Hayes did not like the sound of it either, but he was young, newish and had a healthy respect for the Gipsy Queen.

'I'll examine them in the ambulance if she insists, but if there is any doubt whatsoever, I'm bringing them in,' he insisted and looked unhappy.

As he spoke, the ambulance drew up outside. I dashed towards it with unseemly haste to prevent the unloading of the bodies. As I expected the ambulance men balked and looked ready to start a row, but gave way to Dr Hayes as he quickly ascended the steps to look at the casualties.

'Have a look at that one until I get time to examine him,' he said, indicating what appeared to be the worst specimen.

I felt for his pulse and tried to detect signs of breathing, but it was very much a formality. He couldn't possibly be alive. His whole face had been pushed back into his skull. The nose was upturned and flattened, giving him a grotesquely-jolly appearance, and his skull had snapped at the hairline, exposing the brain. Around his neck hung the shattered remains of his goggles. The arm that I was holding drooped heavily and I noticed it was broken in at least two places.

'Came down Henshaw Hill too fast,' muttered one of the ambulance men, naming a notoriously steep gradient, 'lost control on the bend at the bottom and went smack into one of those flat-sided concrete posts. Must have been killed instantly. We've no idea who they are—no identification on them but we think they're from Glasgow—one's got Glasgow bus tickets and bills in his pocket.'

The other man was in a similar condition, but Dr Hayes, always painstaking and conscientious, seemed extra worried, attempted resuscitation, and examined the bodies for ages, lifting up the dreadfully distorted arms and legs.

'Multiple fractures,' he muttered unnecessarily.

When he finally decided they were dead, the argument started. No, the ambulance men would *not* take the bodies to the public mortuary. They didn't care what our problems were; they had brought the men to hospital and at the hospital they were going to stay. I argued shakily, not having the slightest idea whether I was right, and feeling rather ghoulish about the whole thing anyway. Dr Hayes backed out: it was our problem. The Gipsy Queen appeared suddenly and gave them some real opposition, but they were adamant. Finally, a compromise was reached. They would take them to our mortuary, in the grounds, where they could be laid out later, when time permitted.

A nice young porter and I accompanied the ambulance. When we reached the mortuary, we realized that we had no trolleys on which to put the bodies. The ambulance had to get away so we placed them temporarily on the floor.

'I'll bring the trolleys over,' said the porter. 'Perhaps you can come back later and help me? They haven't been identified yet and it will take the relatives ages to get here from Scotland so we don't have to hurry.'

Smithfield was in a turmoil when I got back and we were desperately trying to catch up when the phone rang again. I cursed. It was the Gipsy Queen—a worried Gipsy Queen.

'Come down here immediately!' she ordered. 'And bring a couple of shrouds with you—hurry!'

I flew down the shiny, echoing corridors, carrying my stiff, white burden.

'They've been claimed quicker than we thought possible. A local young woman phoned the police—her husband and brother, who is on holiday from Scotland, popped out to get some cigarettes and didn't come back. She's on her way to identify them. We can't let her see them on the floor, and in that state!' she exclaimed.

'I'll try to stop her coming but you get over there with the trolleys—*quick!*—and do your best to tidy them up a bit!'

A car was drawing up at Casualty door.

'Quickly!' hastened the Gipsy Queen. 'Out of the front door —run!'

The handsome young porter and I grabbed a trolley each, struggled through the swing doors, down the front steps and started to run up the long path to the mortuary.

It was raining and windy, my cap was coming off and my cloak sliding to one side. I pushed the trolley lengthways but the end kept slewing to one side, bumping into the edge of the path and unloading its contents of shrouds, basins and wads of wool onto the damp grass.

'Try sideways, it's easier to control!' shouted the porter into the wind.

I tried sideways and it was easier for a while. Then the castors, always sticky, jammed and I shot straight over the top. Hysteria was beginning to grip me.

'Hurry, hurry!' yelled my companion.

Suddenly I had one of those moments of extreme mental clarity when one stands outside of oneself and thinks: This is ridiculous—why the hell am I *here* doing *this*? There I was, fleeing in a great panic through the wind and rain, along dark paths in the dead of night, gripping shrouds and tripping over trolleys! A similar feeling had obviously seized the porter for, despite being aware of the tragedy and urgency of our task, we started to giggle helplessly. There was no time to worry about the bogey man as, puffing and panting, we flung open the big doors and pushed in the trolleys.

The bodies were big and very heavy; the floor was slippery with their blood. Lifting them onto the trolleys nearly killed me, but urgency released unknown resources. I put the shrouds on the bodies, then cleaned up their faces while the porter mopped the floor.

Once again I tried to feel sorry for the dead men and to imagine them in real life, with their faces animated and their eyes alive. It bothered me that I couldn't, but it seemed to me that all their personality and human characteristics had gone: they were nothing. It was very disturbing and once again I felt guilty and heartless.

We had just finished when we heard footsteps outside. Suddenly I realized that *I* needed some cleaning up: my apron was soaked with blood. As Sister and the young woman came in I turned my back and slipped outside.

'She insisted on seeing them,' said a young constable. 'We told her someone else could do it but she was adamant.' He shook his head slowly, 'Bloody motor-bikes!'

I moved back quickly as the door opened. Sister and the constable supported the pathetic weeping creature as they led her away. Naturally I was desperately sorry for *her*.

'Hullo, darling,' said a dark-brown voice.

'Phillip?' I was surprised; I'd only seen him a couple of hours before and he knew better than to ring me for a chat at 9 o'clock in the midst of the early night-duty rush. Especially when the Gipsy Queen was liable to loom up at any minute.

'Sorry to bother you, dear,' he said quickly. 'Will you do me a favour?'

'If I can, certainly.' Of course I would. I was pretty gone on Phillip.

'You've had an admission—a guard in a railway accident?' It was a statement rather than a question.

'Yes, as a matter of fact . . .'

'Well, you see, dear—no one else was able to get to him and if I could get a statement it would be quite something for me.'

'A statement? Oh no, I can't let you in!'

'No, silly, you don't have to—just go and ask him what happened. A couple of sentences will do.'

'Really, I shouldn't!'

'No one will know. You can ask him not to tell.'

'Oh, all right then. But if the Gipsy Queen comes, I'll have to pretend you're someone else and ring off.'

'O.K.'

I felt a bit of a fool approaching the man but, although still a little shocked, he was tickled pink by my blushing request.

'Can't tell you much, I'm afraid. I was in the rear coach and there was this big bang and I was thrown to the floor. Didn't see a thing. Don't know what happened really.'

I took the sad news to Phillip.

To my surprise, he was delighted with this seemingly negative statement.

'That's fine, fine,' he enthused. 'Now, what are his injuries?'

'Oh, I don't know if I should . . .'

'Come on—I can get them officially if I want.'

'Well, we don't think it's anything serious. Just shock, lacerations and a query fractured skull—that is, he's going down to X-ray in a minute, just to check.'

Phillip was jubilant and rang off. I felt uneasy at being used so ruthlessly. What if someone found out? But Phillip was quite different from anyone I'd ever met so I had no standards by which to judge him. He was so alive and enthusiastic about everything. Life with him was exciting. Our outings could scarcely be termed exotic. The local bicycle race, boxing and wrestling, chamber music, concerts and Grand Opera performed by the local society. All in pursuit of more and better news. But an interest and enthusiasm in everything transformed them for me, though a certain ghoulish pleasure at other people's misfortune seemed part of a reporter's nature. When all the lights failed during the local company's rendering of *Carmen*, Phillip was delighted. But he was professional enough to hand a rueful bouquet to the reporter on a rival local paper who had headed his piece, 'Pull up for *Carmen*'! Similarly, when I was a bridesmaid and the groom failed to arrive (the cars did not turn up so the poor chap had to thumb a lift to the church, arriving a couple of hours late!), Phillip enthused over his luck and turned it into good copy.

Mr Bernstein had been overjoyed to hear me mention *Carmen* and chamber music; he imagined he'd found a kindred spirit and inveigled me into artistic discussions. I had to flannel like mad to retain my new-found culture-loving image. Oddly enough, Phillip, my Professor Higgins, was also Jewish.

The following evening, an amused railway guard greeted me.

'What's all this in your boy-friend's paper about me having a suspected fractured skull? There's nothing wrong with my head!' he laughed. 'Makes it sound very dramatic, don't it?'

I blushed.

'Well, you did have an X-ray just in case you had fractured your skull. But of course you hadn't,' I hastened to add. 'I suppose it does sound more dramatic put that way.'

Strange things, words, I thought.

The Surgical Registrar's pen hesitated over the notes. 'Go on,' he said.

'Well, I have no definite proof,' I insisted, 'but he'd already complained of severe pain and asked for an injection. Then I saw him again just a split second before he saw me—he put on a display of writhing and moaning just for my benefit and begged for his morphia.'

'Oh dear,' sighed the Registrar and wrote PETHIDINE on the notes in large letters.

'No more morphia—but watch him for withdrawal symptoms!' he said, looking concerned.

'Him' was the young lorry driver who'd been crushed in his cab and we'd been so pleased that we'd pulled him through and killed his pain!

If we'd been less busy I might have noticed his addiction

sooner. The place was getting as bad as Fieldman, I mused, as I paused at last to partake of Mr Latham's coffee and ham sandwiches. No, that wasn't really true. Fieldman was dreadfully overloaded at the moment and Staff Nurse was having his nights off. At supper time, poor Nurse Penfold had looked positively grey at the prospect of being in charge. Fieldman was the only ward which normally had a Staff Nurse *in situ* on nights.

At 12.30 a.m. precisely the phone interrupted my musings. They'd got into the habit of sending Nurse Phipps to theatre and Casualty now that I was in charge. It was the Gipsy Queen all right, but she sounded a little odd.

'Nurse Driscoll, come to Fieldman immediately,' she said slowly and deliberately, '—and take charge.'

CHAPTER XI

Nightmare

My two colleagues could hardly believe their ears when I told them.

'You can't take over *any* ward in the middle of the night! But *Fieldman*! There are over forty patients and it's almost time to start the Night Report! My God, I'm glad it's not me!'

I felt sick. My knowledge of general surgical was quite good but not nearly enough to be in charge—I was only just into my third year.

Sister met me at the ward door—she was not quite as brusque as usual. 'Nurse Penfold was not quite able to cope,' she volunteered, in answer to my puzzled expression. 'She will take over Smithfield.' As she spoke, Staff ushered a weeping Penfold past us and out of the door. 'Come along, I'll show you around the patients. You have an obstruction just about to go down to theatre and a possible perf. coming in. The ward is rather full,' she added mildly, 'and you have several seriously ill patients. We'll concentrate on them first.'

I don't remember much about the rest of that night: memory, or rather lack of it, can be merciful.

In the morning I was greeted by the neat, serene Day Sister who earned my undying gratitude for the serious way she accepted my garbled and quite nonsensical night report and didn't bat an eyelid when the patient total was wrong: I had one over.

'You're not the person I handed over to last night,' she smiled gently. 'I hear it's been rather a bad night.'

I nodded dumbly. My brain was churning with the jobs we should have done, still had to do and might have forgotten. I was incapable of coherent thought and speech.

'Off you go to bed now, have a good sleep,' she shooed me away.

An hour later she caught us in the sluice, finishing off. We knew that the Day Staff couldn't care two hoots about our bad night—they had their own problems. If we left them our work, they'd get behind before they'd even started, they'd hate us, we'd get a bad name and they would not be too fussy about getting done for us. Besides, there was a stigma about not getting done; it suggested one was either lazy or couldn't cope. True, in some cases. But Sister sent us packing with her assurance that the Day Staff would not mind clearing up for us. Oh, dear.

I breathed a long, shuddering sigh of relief when the Staff Nurse returned from his nights off. But I did not return to my Smithfield haven. I remained second in charge and had to take over again on his next dreaded nights off. After a few weeks, he was given a break from nights. We all speculated as to who was going to replace him: few staff nurses would do nights. The replacement turned out to be me.

Actually the Gipsy Queen frightened me almost more than the awful responsibility of the ward. She demanded so much and was so severe if she didn't get it.

My most difficult task was learning names and diagnoses. There were at least half a dozen admissions every day, and I had to learn all the names and diagnoses and be able to match them up with the faces by the time the Gipsy Queen came round at 9 p.m. When dashing past with a bottle of fresh blood for the latest post-op. case, I would point unceremoniously at one of the new ones and say, 'You're Mr Smith and you're a—don't tell me—gastric ulcer!'

They soon caught on that life and death matters took second

place to placating the Gipsy Queen, so when the round started the brighter ones would help me out.

'This is the gastric ulcer,' I would say, as if that were all that was necessary.

'Well, what's his name?' she would exclaim impatiently.

Catching the desperate look in my eye, the patient would jump in innocently with, 'I'm Mr Smith, Sister.'

Other times I'd lead with the name, hoping that the patient would come up with his, 'Can't hold my water' or, 'Stoppage, Sister.'

The good patients also helped to play out the drama of the bedpan-covers. Sister had a mania about bedpan-covers and even insisted that urine bottles should be clothed. But there were never enough to go round and they were always getting lost, so the nurses tore about in the vanguard of 'the round' removing any bare utensils. Sometimes they couldn't manage it and I, knowing there were some in the ward, would steel myself for the expected tirade. But frequently the said objects would miraculously disappear, to emerge later from behind lockers or curtains, or even from under bedclothes.

Snippets of Fieldman's nights stand out from a sea of worry, exhilaration and mental and physical exhaustion:

Dashing into the kitchen for a quick swig of Lucozade to keep me going. No one told me they'd filled an empty Lucozade bottle with Dettol!

My disgust at having to fight to pull a woman out of an insulin coma. She was dying of abdominal cancer complicated by heart disease, hernia and diabetes. Her condition and lack of appetite made diabetic control almost impossible, but we couldn't let her die more easily this way—one can't have insulin coma on a death certificate!

The houseman who, after erecting a succession of drips on patients with difficult veins, grabbed hold of my arm, gazed at the near transparent skin revealing my blood supply traced out like Clapham Junction and exclaimed rapturously, 'What lovely veins you have!'

The reaction of a wife after I had plucked up all my courage to tell her that her husband had died. They were a devoted couple and he died of complications after a reasonably safe operation.

She nodded knowingly. 'That's all right my dear. I knew when I brought him in that he wouldn't come out again—we're Spiritualists you see. I had a message.' She smiled. 'He's still with me!'

I wished she'd passed the message on to us—we'd had a terrible struggle trying to save him!

Wrapping a tray-cloth around the necessary but too bright bed-light of a seriously ill patient who had to be kept under observation. The tray-cloth got singed, so I was ordered to stay up after the full night's duty until 9 a.m. to receive the obligatory berating from Matron. I should have used the blue wrapping paper from cotton-wool rolls.

Becoming more and more irritated at still being treated like a child and at the insulting interference into my private life, considering the immense responsibility I was carrying.

Patients who insisted, 'I can't sleep without my tablets, Nurse,' long after their post-operative drugs should have been needed. They wouldn't countenance large, recognizable codeines, but when given tiny potent-looking vitamin C tablets slept like babes.

.

The above attitude back-firing on us when a patient (who had been an assistant nurse) insisted that the Paraldehyde we gave her (which was administered intramuscularly in unusually large volume and had an extremely distinctive and unpleasant smell) was water!

Waiting visitors beckoning us out of the women's ward when we were frantically busy. Irritably, we ignored them, but eventually went out to find a 'prostate', who had become a little odd of late, standing in the corridor, his wizened, old body clad only in a pyjama top. He was singing loudly and swinging like a lassoo the rubber catheter that was attached to his penis.

Falling asleep at lectures and Mr Prentiss, the lecturing surgeon, saying, 'I realize that you've probably been on nights, Nurse, but this is important!'
But even when I was on days this particular man had only to speak and my eyelids drooped—not through boredom (though he did go on a bit), but due to the positively hypnotic effect of his voice. I drew blood digging my fingers into my arms, trying to fight against the inevitable drowsiness: normally I cannot sleep sitting up.

Being kept very wide awake by a lecturer who should have been a hell-fire and brimstone preacher, with such drama, timing and personality did he issue his message of impending doom. But V.D. was his substitute for the Devil.
'What are women afraid of after casual sexual intercourse?' (dramatic pause) 'Pregnancy!' he would exclaim with disgust, then go on to explain why Spirochaeta pallida and gonococcus were the Devil in disguise compared with dear old honest spermatozoa.
'Syphilis is the Great Imitator!' he would thunder, thumping on the lectern.

His forceful proclamations and examples were not lost on us, and we hastened from each lecture to examine that cold sore on our lip or allergic rash on our tummy with trepidation and renewed respect. Few of us, however, had the time, energy or opportunity to go out and get infected in what he said was the 'real way' everyone caught it. Not the lavatory seat.

A woman patient suddenly growing plump around the neck and face. It turned out to be air in the tissues, a rare post-operative complication. Most odd to press the swelling and feel it move and crackle. Fortunately the air was soon absorbed—after we'd all had a feel.

My brother coming home from Egypt after his two-year stint in the Canal Zone and meeting Jenny (the prettiest girl in the P.T.S.) after they had been pen-friends for a year. Pow! Love at first sight.

An absolutely huge woman being very restless whilst coming out of the anaesthetic.

'Keep an eye on her all the time!' said the Gipsy Queen sternly. Which was a good idea but totally impossible.

I was behind the screens, preparing a man for an emergency obstruction op., when I heard a thunderous crash followed by the sound of breaking glass. It was one of my worst moments when I saw her spreadeagled on the floor, with the smashed drip bottle beside her. The houseman helped us as we struggled to get her back into bed. An extra pair of hands appeared at the vital moment: they belonged to the Gipsy Queen. This was it, I thought, the explosion to end them all.

'There should be someone with her all the time,' she said, after we'd found, to our relief, that no serious damage had been done. But she must have sensed the danger moment: 'I'll send a nurse from Smithfield,' she said mildly. Obviously she did not want another nurse 'not being able to cope' and taken away gibbering.

Sitting straight up in bed during the day and announcing that I must go and look at the drips!

My mounting envy of patients as I tucked them up in bed. The working night was 8 p.m. to 8 a.m. and I was still living at home, so what with never getting off duty on time, over an hour's journey each way and some morning lectures lasting till 11.30 a.m., sleeping time was hopelessly short.

On lecture days, I would sometimes borrow a friend's room to sleep, but the fifth column (the cleaners) soon ratted on me to Home Sister.

Giving woolly instructions to a junior, resulting in her aspirating the wrong patient, and an 'acute abdomen' being sent down for an op. with a stomach full of foul fluid. Which could have been catastrophic if it hadn't been checked in the theatre.

The following morning, after the Gipsy Queen had dessicated me, she related the misdemeanour to my mother. 'I don't know what's the matter with her these days, it's not a bit like her.' (Which amounted to a compliment from the Gipsy Queen).

'She's about to have a nervous breakdown after being on nights for nearly six months,' my mother retorted.

Feeling relieved, then strangely resentful, when a Staff Nurse took over 'my ward' for the last couple of weeks of my night duty. The responsibility had been too terrible for words, but I was hooked.

CHAPTER XII

Migratory Nightingale

I had finally made day-time Casualty, when my parents offered me a trip to Paris for my twenty-first birthday.

My finals were looming large and I was determined that, whatever the result, I would get away from the north. I had become disenchanted with nursing, mainly as a result of that marathon stint on nights and the long months on harrowing Wendover. But I couldn't think of an interesting alternative for which I might be remotely qualified.

In London, en route for Paris, I spied a Woman Police Constable sheltering from the rain in a shop doorway. That's an idea, I thought, a London policewoman! Such was my vocation.

Back home again, I had more finals lectures, including some from my mother, who was now a sister tutor (Jenny, my future sister-in-law was also one of her pupils). I found time, however, to write off to the Metropolitan Police for their enticing brochures.

I filled in their forms, giving minute details of my life and accounting for my whereabouts and behaviour for almost every second of my twenty-one years. I assured them that I was not an epileptic, inclined to insanity, a political extremist nor a sufferer from debilitating period pains.

My first intimation that things were moving, was the familiar summons to Matron's office. She wore an air of pained curiosity.

'Nurse Driscoll,' she sighed, in tones of enduring patience, 'I've had a visit from a Detective Inspector about you!'

But she was clearly impressed by my elevation to such prominence as to warrant a call from a Detective Inspector! For a moment I couldn't think what his purpose could be—surely they wouldn't send him just to enquire whether I'd been a good girl?

'I understand that you have applied to be a *policewoman*!' she stated wonderingly. 'The Detective Inspector was puzzled as to why, after all your training, you should want to leave nursing to be a policewoman?' She uttered the word with obvious distaste. 'I had to confess that I was equally puzzled. Perhaps you could enlighten me?'

She looked hurt. I exercised remarkable restraint (or cowardice) at this juncture, mumbling something about getting in a rut and wanting a change. Matron was not to be fobbed off so easily.

'What does your mother think about it?' she persisted.

'She thinks it's a good idea,' I replied defiantly, but blushed. Such was Matron's powerful and hypnotic personality that I was beginning to feel as if I'd enrolled at the local brothel.

'Well, I *am* surprised that your mother feels like that about it!' Matron said, in a tone which suggested she was nothing of the kind (hadn't she told me before, when objecting to my living out, that my mother spoilt me and gave me too much of my own way?).

Our usual battle of wills ensued but, for once, victory eluded her. My unprecedented move seemed to have thrown her completely and after a few more wondering questions she allowed me to leave, hoping I knew what I was doing.

In the midst of my finals (two sets: a hospital and State Registration—on my 'days off', of course) I took my remaining annual leave and departed to wicked London for the two-day medical and mental examination (or 'nut' and 'gut' as police slang so decorously puts it).

The Metropolitan Police decided that one so sound of wind and limb, able to separate squares from circles, animal from vegetable, write an essay on the industrial development of Burton-on-Trent and 'bull' a board into believing she 'loved people' (ghastly indiscriminating phrase) was fit to be a guardian of the hub of the Universe.

My application and acceptance caused something of a sensation throughout the hospital. No one had ever taken such a decision when they were (hopefully) just about to qualify. Renouncing one's vows was startling enough, but *going to London*. I should mention that most northerners regard 'the South' as another country and are deeply suspicious of that alien land. London is all right for cup finals and all that goes with them (wink, wink, nudge, nudge) but to want to *live* there is slightly immoral, or insane, or both.

'What does your mother say about you going to London?' was the fascinated question, persistently posed.

'She thinks it's a good idea,' I replied airily, whence they retired, shocked at such parental abandonment.

The young Australian Assistant-Surgeon now on Wendover (where I was working yet again) couldn't understand my wanting to become an object of such contempt and loathing, and was determined to save me.

'You'll only go and marry a policeman,' he said. 'Stay in this and you could end up with a surgeon [Big deal!]. Look, if you want a change, emigrate to Australia. I'll give you some introductions.'

Australians were always trying to get me to go to Australia: it may be pertinent that they were usually resident here.

The senior nursing staff took it all as a personal affront. Whenever I was late, they would say, 'You'll have to change your ways when you're in the Police, my girl. They won't stand for this slackness. You're in for a shock when you find out what discipline really is!'

And suddenly it was time to leave St Margaret's and all that it meant: the excitement of being right at the heart of things; the feeling I was missing Life; the instant comradeship I still felt when meeting one of my old P.T.S. classmates; the hatred that a colleague who wouldn't pull her weight could engender in me; the vain thrill of laundry day when I emerged from the staff room feeling splendid in the supremely flattering, fresh striped dress, crackling snowy apron, rigid collar and perkiest of perky caps; the cosiness of working on a ward where I 'belonged' and was therefore greeted extravagantly after the shortest absence; the social kudos bestowed by our profession; the ever-increasing feeling of social inadequacy when trying to converse with people who read papers and had interests and activities outside their jobs; the irksome discipline that made me want to scream and break out, only I hadn't the time and was too tired anyway; wondering what the younger nurses were coming to—no discipline and not of the calibre we had been in our day; the patients who became coy and laboriously engineered conversations with 'their nurse' when I served tea during visiting time; the utter peace and suspension of reality when walking the deserted, shiny corridors in the dead of night; the demanding, 'Nurse!'—irritating, exhausting, yet making me feel important; the persistent poverty which made me want some unattainable pretty thing with a desperation quite out of proportion to its worth (young London nurse with the right accent and hailing from the Home Counties, don't tell me this is not so. You're a different breed and can be let out of your cage of poverty and the daily grind by those rich indulgent parents); my deliberately developed air of confidence; the growing bossiness in my manner; the bond felt with patients with whom one had shared the struggle for life. And so many more confused memories and mixed feelings.

As with most things I do, my nursing was good in parts. I could be exceptionally capable at times, then let myself down by some appallingly stupid error, or by exposing evidence of an astonishing gap in my knowledge—some information that my odd brain had rejected or refused to grasp.

In many ways being a Reluctant Nightingale was a pretty awful experience yet even now I have only to catch the evocative smell of antiseptic, or see the self-important bustle of a busy casualty department, and I am seized by a very potent nostalgia.

Those of our class that were left—a handful only—took jobs as Staff Nurses at St Margaret's or other hospitals. Others became District Nurses. Jenny married my brother. Recently, after undergoing an appendicectomy she said to me:

'Hey, you know how we used to tell patients off for hobbling about all bent up, and say, "Goodness, you've only had an appendicectomy, not a major op." Well, I was determined to stand up straight after mine but, my God—it hurts!'

On the day I entered Peel House to commence my police training, I received a telegram from my mother, 'Congratulations—S.R.N.' I've scarcely used the designation since, except on a few rare occasions when I wished to give a little extra respectability to my signature. And I do that less and less as time passes, in case people start going on about their bad legs and internal troubles or expect me to practise first aid.

I was settling down quite well to being a policewoman, but couldn't seem to get to work on time.

'I don't know,' commented our Woman Inspector despairingly, 'I'm sure they didn't allow you to be late when you were a nurse!'

'No, Sister—I mean Inspector,' I agreed.

Epilogue

But seriously, what was wrong with hospital nursing?

The administration for one thing. It is an error to assume that a good nurse will necessarily make a good administrator or enjoy being one. It is interesting to note that Florence Nightingale's principal genius lay in administration. As Cecil Woodham-Smith pointed out in her excellent biography, *Florence Nightingale*: 'It was not as an angel of mercy that she was asked to go to Scutari . . . her mission was to be an administrator.'

In 1963 the Ministry of Health admitted that job definition, selection and training for senior posts was in a mess when they appointed the Salmon Committee on Senior Nursing Staff Structure. Their report in 1967 recognized: that senior nursing staff tend 'to interfere in ward matters more than they ought to', often satisfying their own needs rather than those of the patients or ward sisters; that managerial positions should be seen to be of equal importance to the patients as actual nursing; 'that some highly skilled nurses do not have the managerial capacities that are necessary for the most senior positions'; that 'nurses in top management need, most of all, well-developed managerial skills'.

Amongst other things they recommended were: standardization of job descriptions; more delegation of authority and trivial tasks; early recognition of administrative ability which should then be encouraged and trained (at the time of the report only 212 out of 2,045 matrons in England and Wales had taken any kind of administration course); the expanding of alternative avenues for the advancement of the skilled but not admin.-minded nurse, such as the charge of a specialized unit where her skill can be used but patient contact maintained, or participation in an expanded and upgraded tutorial side.

The Matron of St Margaret's was by far the best I came across. She did have intelligence, administrative ability and was by and large fair-minded. But she was middle-aged and a spinster and therefore remote from our world. She obviously found it difficult both to acquire funds to improve nursing conditions and to throw off the tradition mania that was supported by her other senior staff and which had been instilled into her.

Tradition. Tradition it was which demanded I go to see Matron to book my holiday period, go again before I went on holiday to tell her I was going, write to her whilst away to say I was coming back, then formally report back when I had started again. The latter had presumably not been noted by the Assistant Matron to whom I had checked in for duty, nor by the ward sister. All such visits were made during my coffee-break, so often meant no break and no coffee. It was merely courtesy, we were told. Merely a waste of time. Sickness demanded the same procedure, except that one couldn't book the period beforehand; no wonder they got so upset about it.

Among nursing's worst enemies is that section of the general public which delights in the 'angel of mercy' and 'it's a vocation' myth and speak in hushed tones of 'the sick', as though they were a separate race, not just ordinary people under stress. Such people imagine that overwork, poor pay and bad conditions are quite acceptable because, as they say with a sweet, idealistic light shining in their eyes, 'They don't do it for the money, do they?'

Nurses do the job because it's interesting (interesting jobs for women are still few and far between: I know—I've worked in an employment agency!), carries status and they like to feel they are doing a useful job, just like everyone else. They would like more money and better conditions, just like everyone else. Unfortunately, some nurses help to sustain this silly but flattering 'saint' image. They're not so saintly to each other and I can only speak from experience when I say that those who professed any serious vocation were certainly no better and often a lot worse than the others; worse, because often they became too involved with individuals or were hypocrites or just too juvenile to identify their own motives.

But the public must have their whiter-than-white saints and their blacker-than-black villains (I've been a 'saintly' nurse and a 'brutal, power-crazed' police officer, which makes me pretty peculiar), and woe betide you if you join a group which has been nominated for either position and you try to kick it. Police officers, though I feel you won't believe a word of it, are much nicer to work with (not just the men) *because* their conditions are better.

Pay and, in many hospitals, conditions have improved, though they still vary considerably. The three-shift system is more widely used instead of the Victorian two-shift which I worked; weekly lectures have largely been superseded by a couple of weeks in training school from time to time; employment of more domestic staff and ward orderlies and the modernization of wards and equipment are freeing the nurses to nurse. But from my contacts in the profession I gather that there are still too many hospitals where improvements are hindered both by lack of money and by the timid, unintelligent mind which finds tradition safer than reform.

Nurses have become tired of being the nation's favourite martyrs and are now fighting for their right to better conditions. Not being able to strike (morally) does hinder them of course. But the main complaint is still as constant as ever: 'the way "they" treat us'; 'the way "they" speak to us'. 'They' of course being the seniors from Staff Nurse upwards.

'As if we're not even human.'

'They want our whole lives.'

'Nobody cares about us. If we go sick we're either malingering or it's our own fault because we've been staying out late at nights.'

To me this is the whole crux of the matter. Tradition and attitudes within the nursing profession itself. So what can be done?

Growing female emancipation should aid general confidence and lessen the aggressiveness. Younger women now being promoted are reported to be usually better than their older predecessors, though not always. The Salmon Committee admitted to some traditionalism and put its faith in education, re-organization, delegation of authority and the establishment of more middle-management admin. people. Well, it will be a few years yet before one can judge the effects of these. They are being adapted gradually, but naturally there are teething troubles.

I'm glad to see many more admin. courses are being attended but they tend to be of the shorter two- or three-month variety; enrolment is down for the Royal College of Nursing's twelve-month course which gives more time for concentration on personnel handling. But one nurse educator concerned about this problem admitted dishearteningly that there was no evidence that admin.-course trained staff had any better record for personnel handling. 'We can't change their personalities and something seems to happen to nurses during their three-year training which makes them behave like this on promotion.' (Getting their own back perhaps?) Also: 'There is a grave shortage of first-class people at the top.'

So my last word is for those unenlightened members of the senior staff. For goodness' sake stop saying, 'the patient comes first' in that smug, self-righteous manner. Student nurses are people too and by not treating them as such you are showing your own ignorance. It is the patient who suffers in the end by being tended by unhappy, overworked nurses and finally—because no-one wants the job—by not being nursed at all.

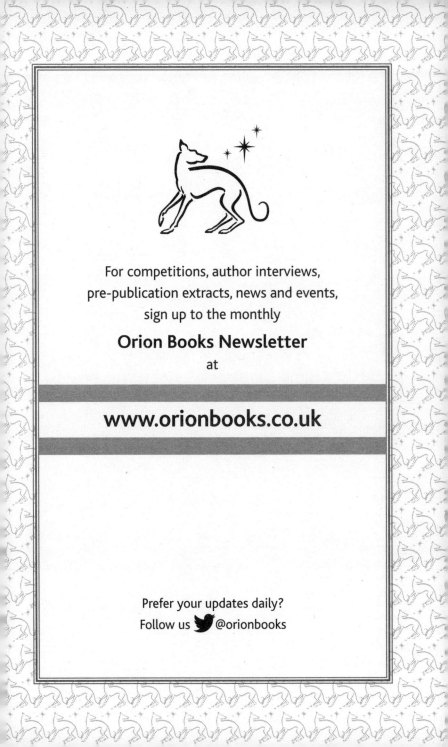

For competitions, author interviews,
pre-publication extracts, news and events,
sign up to the monthly

Orion Books Newsletter

at

www.orionbooks.co.uk

Prefer your updates daily?
Follow us 🐦 @orionbooks